THE COMPLETE GUIDE TO LONG COVID-19

How To Survive & Thrive Your Pathway To Recovery

GRETA STEINER

CONTENTS

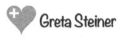

GET THE EXTRAS!

R.I.S.E. Protocol®
Diet Plans & Nutrition Guide

Facebook Group
to return to health

By Greta Steiner

It's totally free with no strings attached,
so for instant access, just sign up at:

ts-publishing.com/gretasteiner

INTRODUCTION

"*To be honest, I was terrified of this virus, not for me but for my loved ones that I live with that I could possibly infect. I live with my mother who has health issues, so I went straight into isolation. It felt like a tractor had driven over me, I was in pain and felt constantly tired. Even after the 14 days I continued feeling tired after doing the simplest of household tasks. I visited my doctor and dietitian who helped me change my lifestyle. This was where I learned about long COVID-19 and that I was unlucky to have had it. I wasn't going to let this get the better of me, so I exercised, focused on my health and tried to get back to normalcy. It was hard, but after two months of fighting I did it. I wasn't going to be another statistic - I beat long COVID-19 and I want my story to be the inspiration to others that you can do it to.*" *– Shaakirah Agulhas*

The above statement should provide much concern as the effects of COVID-19 are real. We are witnessing the repercussions every single day, in the interactions we have with our family, friends and coworkers. The virus is affecting people, it is causing their early demise, with those that have been cured presenting with symptoms that exist for months after the infection. The COVID-19 pandemic has resulted in much pain, sadness and hopelessness. You may have lost someone due to COVID-19, or even survived the virus yourself. However, it doesn't matter which part of the spectrum you are on, the key information regarding what happens after being infected with COVID-19 is what is present in this book, enabling you to focus on your own recovery.

What the quote further points us to is the concept of "long COVID-19." This term is the literal definition of the words, referring to an illness that is present in individuals who are reporting lasting effects even once having retested negative for COVID-19. These symptoms that are experienced can range from a continuous fever, to that of newly developed joint pain. Research shows that two-fifths of patients that presented with long COVID had a worsened quality of life. A study performed by the *Journal of the American Medical Association* showed that up to 87% of patients discharged after testing positive for COVID-19, experienced at least one symptom that remained for a minimum time period of 60 days post-infection. What is a bit more concerning is that 55% of the 87% that exhibited prolonged symptoms, had three or more symptoms for at least a 60-day period. With that being said, one in ten patients reported feeling sick for three weeks or more.

In order to allow the interaction and support for individuals that have long COVID-19, support groups have aided in people's anxiety drastically decreasing as many believe they are the only people who have a prolonged set of symptoms. What healthcare institutes are now implementing, is the establishment of studies that follow patients who have had COVID-19 for at least a year. This is done to see if there are any urgent long-term effects that need to be considered when initiating, altering and/or potentiating a patient's treatment.

Mental health has affected nearly everyone during the pandemic. Many have been under strict lockdown regulations, resulting in feelings of isolation and detachment from the happenings of the world. Even if you haven't directly been impacted by the COVID-19 pandemic, nothing says that you will not be affected. You may even want to take precautionary measures and learn all you can about the coronavirus however, one must be careful regarding what information is read. With all the hearsay that is making its way around the web, this book has the function of breaking down the myths of COVID-19 and long COVID-19, telling you the truth about the pandemic, but most importantly, providing information on how to look after yourself and the people in your circles, during and post-infection.

As an individual of the general public you probably have so many questions but not enough answers. This is where I come in. There is an abundance of information regarding studies and testing modalities within the COVID-19 domain. However, with the newly coined development of long COVID-19, the research surrounding this is both intriguing and fascinating. Having done research into the medical jargon to understand the core modalities of long COVID-19 development, I am able to string together vital information about long COVID-19. This includes providing tools that will aid you on the pathway of recovery, applicable pre, during and post-infection with COVID-19.

The road to recovery does not stop when your COVID-19 test result comes back negative. A virus, especially one that has the capacity to develop symptoms after initial infection, whilst still testing negative, may take weeks to months in order for its effects to be completely overcome. This does not only refer to physical effects, but places emphasis on the mental, emotional and social impact the virus has on our everyday functioning and interactions with others.

COVID-19 is a complex and real virus, affecting livelihoods without discrimination. In this book we will be focusing on the practical steps towards coping with "Long COVID-19" (i.e., the symptoms associated during the recovery period after you have been cured of COVID-19), which will include the therapies and treatment available, as well as the nutrition and supplementation necessary for you to have an immune system that prevents further infection. A holistic approach will be taken, whereby we provide examples of good mindfulness and wellbeing practices, coupled with steps that will aid in managing your anxiety during this difficult and confusing time.

The primary intent of this book is to alleviate your symptoms in a manner that you understand and are comfortable with. Furthermore, we want to make sure that you understand where you can obtain correct information, that is not hidden behind a facade of false statistics. With the effect of long COVID-19 on one's mental health, we want to alleviate that burden by providing you with mindfulness techniques that ensure you do not succumb to the fear that can be associated with long COVID-19.

The media has allowed a stigma to be placed on those that are infected with COVID-19. However, what they don't do is shed insight on the importance of supportive therapy and how altering your lifestyle in a healthy manner can allow you to deal with long COVID-19 more effectively. We see this type of stigma with those that have been infected with HIV/AIDS. However, one can learn to live with COVID-19 and long COVID-19. Practical aspects which include how to run your house while you are in the recovery phase, as well as questions such as, "when do you return to work," and "how do you interact with others," will all be answered in this book.

If one is able to establish adequate and effective preventative measures, the impact that the virus will have on the livelihood of humanity will be drastically decreased. The supposed secrets regarding COVID-19 and long COVID-19 will be unearthed and critically discussed, allowing peace of mind and will decrease any anxiety or fear that you, or someone you know, may have.

1

Long COVID-19 Secrets Revealed

Contents:

CHAPTER 1

THE HIDDEN EPIDEMIC

"Love and a cough cannot be hid."
–George Herbert

COVID-19 has become a buzzword across the globe over the past few months. Having started in China, within a period of fewer than six months, COVID-19 was quickly crossing the globe, leading to the World Health Organization (WHO) classifying the SARS-CoV-2 (scientific name for COVID-19 as it can present with sudden acute respiratory syndrome) virus as a pandemic in March 2020. Although there is still no direct answer as to where the initial infection from Wuhan, China came from, there have been many absurd conspiracy theories that some have tried to base on facts. What we can assure you, is that COVID-19 did not come from an individual eating a bat.

For many of us, this is the first pandemic we have lived through, and may not be aware of the greater effects a pandemic may have. With this we aren't referring to the economic impact, or the alteration in our social lives. We are referring to the existence of a hidden epidemic. In the case of COVID-19, the hidden epidemic is the post-viral symptoms that are associated with long COVID-19. The reason we say it is hidden, is because once one is tested negative for COVID-19, they are removed from the system with minimal follow-up. Thus, the intensity for long COVID-19 acknowledgment is shrouded by the initial burst of media and urgency that arrived with the COVID-19 pandemic.

Naturally, due to different healthcare systems, some with national health insurance and others without, countries reacted in different manners to the virus. An example of this would be Trinidad and Tobago that implemented strict lockdown procedures after hitting a daily infection rate of 80 new infections per day. Retrospectively, there are countries like that of South Africa that have started opening up interprovincial travel and their economy after the number of new cases decreased from approximately 14,000 per day, to that of approximately 4,000 per day. Each government has different views on this pandemic, and are implementing changes, measures and contingency plans as they see fit.

To see how countries were affected differently, we will take a look at the different approaches towards COVID-19 that these countries instituted. China reported the first case of COVID-19 on the 31st December 2019 (a fantastic way to enter into 2020), with the city of Wuhan being placed under quarantine late January 2020. The Chinese government responded by rapidly building new hospitals, whilst placing more stringent restrictions on the freedom to express views across media platforms. This was with the main intent of containing the spread of misinformation and fake news.

Italy was devastated by COVID-19 primarily because its population is largely composed of the elderly. Even though Italy is seen as having one of the most advanced healthcare systems in the world, the rapid rate at which infections were occurring exposed potholes within the system, overwhelming and almost collapsing the healthcare system. Italy's government could not respond fast enough however, they did show that through implementing strict social distancing measures coupled with extensive testing protocols and proactive tracing, the COVID-19 outbreak could be contained.

A country that was heavily affected was South Africa. Due to the large financial inequality present, along with a high burden of HIV/AIDS, diabetes, hypertension and tuberculosis, the government needed to act fast. With the South African Defence Force (SADF) being deployed to ensure rules of lockdown are adhered to, residents and organizations were forcefully removed from premises and jailed for not adhering to government protocols.

Resources across countries and communities were stretched to limits that we had never seen. With there being rumors across the globe stating that there was to be a shortage of toilet paper, the news was flooded with images and videos of people loading up and to an extent hoarding large amounts of toilet paper. This along with the sudden shortages of hand sanitizers, disinfectants and clean water to wash hands, had many around the world fearing the reality that could have been them contracting COVID-19. The disparity between the rich and the poor grew immensely, with those that don't have access to adequate nutrition having their immune systems negatively affected, increasing their chances of contracting COVID-19.

However, with all of the negative press that this pandemic brought, there were many positives. One included the hike in innovation and the need to find alternative solutions to work remotely whilst not compromising on the quality and amount of work that could be completed. Many schools and universities shifted to a new era of online learning which proved to have its own challenges, yet allowing students to work at their own pace and in the comfort of their own homes.

There have been multiple instances of people needing to source and fend for themselves, focussing on establishing a standard manner of living that allows optimal human functioning. However, for those that were not as privileged to interact and obtain food, medicine, money for masks and preventative equipment, faith in humanity was restored. We saw clothing lines converting their manufacturing facilities into solely creating masks for the public, communities came together to create food parcels for the less fortunate, with medical care (including psychological and psychiatric consultations) being shifted to an online platform. Accessibility was altered in terms of service delivery however, this did not alter the resultant outcome in terms of quality of health without the restrictions that COVID-19 has imposed.

It is human nature that we are able to interact on a social level. Remove this and we find ourselves falling into a cycle of depression, anxiety and uncertainty. This cycle would typically have resulted in a decrease in work ethic, heightened stress and biologically a weaker immune system. In order to explain this and solidify understanding, we shall focus on some human biology. When we are stressed, our body produces cortisol, a stress hormone that enables us to cope with our thoughts and external surroundings. However, a negative effect on this is that cortisol weakens our body's immunity towards infections. This means that it doesn't matter how well you eat, whether you take copious amounts of vitamins, and exercise daily, stress will hinder your health, affecting your response to the COVID-19 virus as well as opportunistic infections both whilst being infected with COVID-19, and post-infection.

The COVID-19 infection itself can be overcome - it is possible! Many patients are asymptomatic (i.e., do not show any physical signs of infection) which shows that many individuals have had the virus, and lived their lives normally without any hindrances. Many patients who have tested positive for COVID-19 reported that they felt fatigued, short of breath, as well as lethargic for a varying period of time once they retested and had a negative result.

A real-life example is Paul Garner, who is a professor at the Liverpool School of Tropical Medicine. Having contracted COVID-19 in March 2020, he spent a total of seven weeks in a constant state of severe exhaustion coupled with emotions that were on the extreme ends of the depression and anxiety spectrum. Paul had long COVID-19. His symptoms shifted from being dizzy to developing an upset stomach, pins and needles in his extremities and a ringing in his ears. These symptoms persisted for weeks, coming and going with varying levels of severity. There is no definitive trajectory for the

COVID-19 pandemic however, understanding the impact that long COVID-19 has on one's life will allow for measures to be instituted that drastically decrease the impact that long COVID-19 can have on your life.

The number of individuals that are reporting the prolongation of their symptoms are rising. The main complaint that is given is that there is a change in their symptoms from when they tested positive for COVID-19, to that of when they tested negative. With the chances of them already having traversed into long COVID-19 territory, their approach to their symptoms would need to change. This probes us to ask the question regarding the possible long-term effects that COVID-19 has. Up to 45% of those that test positive for COVID-19 will not show any physical symptoms of infection, whereas 1% of infections will present as life-threatening pneumonia that will require ventilation and hospitalization.

Long COVID-19 is a serious issue, one which all governments should be researching. At the end of the day, the effects of long COVID-19 will impact the ability of those to work, the earning potential of the country, the Gross Domestic Profit (GDP) as well as the degree of trade that occurs between countries. However, with the government implementing support groups, patient self-help forms the cornerstone of empowering people to take action for themselves and on their own terms. One needs to provide people who have had COVID-19 with the tools, knowledge and empowerment that allows a shift in their mindset towards overcoming their current situations. What this will do, is allow their body to recuperate and fight the lingering symptoms post-infection, whilst still allowing time for mindfulness practices.

When you decide that you are no longer going to be a victim of a virus, your consciousness acknowledges this decision. We tend to discount the effect that our brain has on how we feel, when in actual fact it is what gives us the energy to overcome obstacles.

CHAPTER 2

PERSONAL STORIES

"Knowledge comes, but wisdom lingers."
—Alfred, Lord Tennyson

In order for us to put long COVID-19 into perspective, it is imperative that we provide you with some real-life stories of individuals that suffered through long COVID-19 and survived.

The story of Chrystal is a very typical presentation of how one would generally think about COVID-19. She came into contact with COVID-19 via a coworker from her husband's office. Many, like Chrystal, developed a level of anxiety that resulted in halting all external activities and confining family members to learn and work from home. Chrystal's husband started to develop a scratchy throat which did not escalate any further, with her entire family remaining in the house and not having any contact with the outside world, primarily due to fear of contracting the virus, but also to prevent possible transmission to the elderly that are at risk. Like many, Chrystal and her family enjoyed the first few days of lockdown, only for her to complain that she cannot smell when cooking fish one night. She hopped onto Google to do some research and discovered that losing your sense of smell was supposedly a symptom associated with younger asymptomatic patients. She believed that was the extent of her infection. Unfortunately, 14 weeks later she was housebound, gasping for air when doing the slightest bit of physical movement, as well as having instances of pain that made her think her kidneys or liver were failing.

With Chrystal now believing the worst has passed, her sense of smell returned, only to be substituted with gut issues that were typical with food poisoning. She started developing severe bouts of shortness of breath, only for an x-ray to inform her she had developed pneumonia (note that we are still post-infection). She felt tingling and numbness in her right arm and leg, which caused her to rush to the emergency department with the thought that she had a stroke. She was sent home and told she should feel better in two weeks. However, leading up to the two-week mark her headaches escalated in frequency and severity. She struggles to do housework and look after her children because the slightest movements cause immense fatigue. Chrystal implemented all the protective measures, washing hands regularly and maintaining social distancing. She remains rather sick, but believes she is getting better day by day. She believes that healthcare professionals need to understand that there are long-term implications of COVID-19 that is harboring normal family function. Chrystal looks forward to the days when she feels energetic and lively again, so that she can play and interact with her kids.

We can see that there is a very significant and severe impact that

COVID-19 can have on an individual, their daily functioning, as well as the truth that long COVID-19 does exist. We have been able to observe the effects and views from someone who has their own family however, what about those that are in the lower age ranges? To show these effects, we have the story of Shaun and his experience with long COVID-19.

Shaun is a 20-year-old male that is as fit as a fiddle, not having any underlying health conditions that he is aware of. On March 13th, Shaun (who is from the UK) started feeling symptoms that were related to infection with the COVID-19 virus. Having felt this way two weeks before the UK went into a state of lockdown, he remained cautious, staying at home and keeping himself busy with his studies.

Like many others, Shaun cannot say for certain where he contracted the virus from however, believes it was most probably an interaction with a food delivery service. However, what Shaun did which many people did not think of, is having limited contact with other individuals during COVID19's incubation period. Shaun's journey with COVID-19 is different from your typical course as he started to develop pain in his lungs, fever and chills. But, because Shaun did not present with any shortness of breath he was not allowed to be tested, despite having varied symptoms from day to day which included headaches, confusion, chest pains and sleep apnoea.

Where Shaun's situation became direr is due to the lack of support or aid that was received by the UK government and healthcare systems. Based on his age as well as not having any previous or underlying conditions, his symptoms were said to be due to severe anxiety.

Although he had suffered from anxiety before, he knew that this was different. Shaun knew that he was feeling unwell.

Shaun's symptoms persisted for longer than six weeks, with the healthcare system labeling him as having post-viral effects and symptoms. The treatment that he received was being told to go home and let the virus' effects take its course. Shaun made the decision to join a COVID-19 recovery group so that he was able to connect with others who were going through similar situations that he was. It was even after going for more tests with his General Practitioner (GP), that even after they were all normal, he began to enter a cycle of feeling absolutely horrible, then better, then absolutely horrible again.

Shaun has suffered from chest pains, weakness, headaches, nausea, bouts of diarrhea and vomiting every single day. This is after he had felt ill for more than two months after the initial symptoms of COVID-19 started. From what we can tell by comparing this story to the one of Chrystal's is that long COVID-19 does not discriminate–it has the ability to affect people from all different walks of life. We see this especially with our next story from Meghan. Meghan has kept a detailed journal of the times in which she felt ill, when her symptoms got worse, as well as the true effects of long COVID-19, especially how it negatively affects your quality of life.

Meghan had a feeling from the beginning of the pandemic that there was going to be a high chance she contracted it as her mom worked with international students and lockdown regulations had yet to be implemented. Meghan did everything a worried parent and daughter would do. She bought a thermometer to monitor everyone's temperature, vitamin supplements for their immune systems, copious amounts of hand sanitizer, as well as biodegradable antiviral wipes. One would say that Meghan had been over-prepared and would not contract COVID-19.

However, once Meghan's daughter started to develop a cough, she started to worry. She did what any parent would do and removed her child from school. Meghan was then called by her daughter's school and told that it was irrational to keep her daughter from going to school when there were other kids present in class that had also developed a cough. This already showed the disregard that the school and government systems had in acknowledging the seriousness of the COVID-19 pandemic.

The next morning, Meghan developed a fever and felt a burning sensation in her chest and airways. She called the healthcare services and was clinically diagnosed with COVID-19. It was that same night that she lost consciousness twice, found herself gasping for breath, as well as feeling delusion about where she was. It was then that Meghan's entire family went into isolation. The post-viral effects for Meghan persisted, even once everyone else in the family felt healthy. She had terrible headaches that felt like migraines, neck pain that didn't allow her to sleep adequately, eye pain, as well as a burning sensation in her lungs that prevented her from being able to sleep at night.

Meghan then felt well on the seventh day since she experienced COVID-19 symptoms. However, this feeling of elation was short-lived, as she experienced severe headaches and neck pain that warranted a visit to the emergency department of her local hospital, only days after she believed she was cured. Meghan then went home and continued to develop more severe symptoms which included blood-shot eyes, a crawling skin sensation, as well as a tingling sensation in her tongue and lips. Four months later and the symptoms are still present, with no sign of getting better anytime soon. Long COVID-19 is real, and the government, society and the healthcare systems need to acknowledge this and treat accordingly.

With the stories that we have read of in this chapter, it is clear that long COVID-19 is real, and that it is diminishing the quality of lives of individuals across the world. Research and management protocols need to be put in place whereby treatment methodologies are created and implemented. This seems to be a challenging approach, especially because it seems as if patients who exhibit post-viral symptoms, all present with varying types of symptoms.

If we are able to establish the root cause of the post-viral symptoms, we may be able to sufficiently and effectively treat these patients, allowing them to live a normal life. Thus, using the information and knowledge in these stories, along with the research regarding long COVID-19, a greater approach towards self-help measures can be instituted and reinforced. Not only will this decrease the burden on already overburdened healthcare systems, but it will also allow those affected to take ownership of their condition.

CHAPTER 3

SYMPTOMS

"Our emotional symptoms are precious sources of life and individuality."
—*Thomas More*

Long COVID-19 is associated with being a post-viral illness. To break this down into simpler terms, it is seen as a specific group of symptoms that present after complete cure of a viral infection. Some specific viral infections may have completely different symptoms as a part of their post-viral illness presentation however, for the sake of this book we will be tackling those that focus specifically with long COVID-19. In this specific section we are going to explain the symptoms that are associated with long COVID-19, as well as be able to classify the severity of these symptoms. The classification of the severity becomes important, especially when you need to draw the line between continuing self-help care and needing the expertise of a healthcare practitioner.

EXPECTED SYMPTOMS

Many of the symptoms that someone with long COVID-19 will experience, will differ in severity, all of them having strategies to manage them in a prompt and effective manner. What is important to note in this section is that one needs to know when further self-help becomes futile, leading to professional help needing to be sought out.

MIND FOG

This specific form of fog is also known as "brain fog" in other forms of literature, which needs to be remembered, especially if you are going to be doing your own research on how you are feeling. Although mind fog is not seen as a medical condition, it in its own entity consists of its own subset of symptoms. These symptoms will include you being unable to recall memories (both recent and past), an immense difficulty in concentration, leading to a severe form of mental fatigue. Typically, the first sign that one may in fact have mind fog, is that the person feels that their thought processes have become fuzzy, feeling a lack of sharpness in being able to think of finer details.

A person with mind fog will not feel like themselves, and will express not being able to think clearly. With someone who is experiencing other symptoms due to long COVID-19, mind fog may develop as a sign of a change in one's diet, as well as the initiation of any recent medication for a chronic condition. One way to know to delineate whether the mind fog is due to an illness or to personal lifestyle is by simply getting more sleep. The main cause of mind fog is when you don't sleep enough. Thus, the treatment is patient-specific and based on causality. If one feels that they are unable to find the cause, and that self-help regulation of sleeping patterns does not work, a visit to a physician is then warranted for core analysis and aid.

BURNING LUNGS

For individuals that have a history of heart conditions, having a feeling of your lungs burning can be a frightening experience. With burning lungs, there are two possible causes. One could be that your airways are inflamed, making the act of breathing feel as if your lungs are on fire, or two, that you have chest pain that is mimicking the sensation of burning lungs. Long COVID-19 has the potential to cause a feeling of burning lungs in a variety of different ways. This includes heartburn/acid reflux, problems in your gastrointestinal system (the passage from your mouth to your anus), muscle or bone injuries that are more prevalent due to the effects that long COVID-19 has on the body, panic attacks due to heightened levels of anxiety, lung health issues, as well underlying heart diseases that have yet to be diagnosed.

What we tend to see is that those with long COVID-19 that have burning lungs post-viral infection, had pneumonia during their initial infection. Burning lungs is a serious symptom and will need the professional expertise of a healthcare professional in order for the root cause to be obtained. However, in the case of long COVID-19, a complete medical history coupled with blood work, an electrocardiogram and chest x-rays will need to be done in order for the root cause of the burning lungs to be identified and applicable treatment to be promptly initiated.

In terms of self-care for burning lungs, there are some possible remedies that may work to alleviate the pain. These remedies include lying down and taking slow, deep breaths whilst gently massaging the painful area. To see whether the burning lungs are due to heartburn/acid-reflux one can take an antacid as well as drink a glass of water. Surgical interventions may need to happen depending on what the causative instance was upon medical examination. The important aspect that people with long COVID-19 need to understand is when they should see a doctor. If you feel a sudden and intense burning sensation in your chest, an intense pressure or pain in the center of the chest, chest pain and burning that gets worse and does not improve with home remedies, a visit to the emergency unit of your nearest healthcare facility is warranted as life-saving treatment may need to be initiated.

PINS AND NEEDLES

This specific symptom refers to a tingling sensation that is typically felt at the tips of your extremities, so in your fingers and toes. Although this is a fairly common symptom, it can be the first sign associated with a more complex disease process. It is important to mention that the feeling of pins and needles can be classified as severe, episodic or chronic. It typically accompanies muscle wasting as well as nerve damage—characteristically associated with viral infections like that of the post-viral illness of long COVID-19. However, some people may see there being a more prevalent appearance of this specific symptom if they have previously diagnosed chronic conditions, for example, diabetes.

If not treated adequately, the pins and needles in the extremities (more commonly called peripheral neuropathy) will result in decreased mobility and possible disability. A great advantage regarding the nerves in our extremities is that if the nerve cells have not been destroyed, they can regenerate. Some self-help treatment modalities that can be adopted include that of maintaining your optimal weight for your height, age and gender, following an exercise program that has been approved by a doctor, eating a balanced diet, limiting (or completely removing) alcohol consumption, and ensuring that you stop smoking.

Where the possibility of needing to see a healthcare professional comes in, is that if there is a vitamin deficiency that is being caused by long COVID-19, vitamin levels will need to be established. Seeing as there is a large possibility that a vitamin deficiency can cause pins and needles, with their normal levels being achieved through supplementation, this symptom can be alleviated.

BREATHLESSNESS

This specific symptom is directly related to the sensation of being short of breath, or alternatively having difficulty in breathing normally. Although it is also a common symptom, it can be very distressing to experience. Once a patient develops long COVID-19 there is a concomitant effect on the lungs, which may be potentiated if the respiratory system was affected during the initial COVID-19 infection. It is typical that one's breathlessness is worsened by doing exercise or when undergoing physical exertion. This is why it is so important to see a healthcare practitioner as your breathlessness will be graded, which will have an impact on the type of treatment regimen that you will be given. There are four main manners which you can develop breathlessness, especially with long COVID-19. The post-viral illness may result in a decrease in the amount of oxygen that is in your bloodstream, decreasing the ability of your lungs to expand, which will hinder the removal of carbon dioxide from your bloodstream.

Well, now that the biology lessons are done, let us look at some of the treatment modalities for people who develop breathlessness as a symptom of their long COVID-19. Depending on the severity of breathlessness you may need to be given morphine to slow down your rate of breathing. Oxygen is given, with many people benefitting from it. Medication may also be given (these are called bronchodilators) as it will aid in the opening up of your airways. Although, treatment may not necessarily have to occur in a hospital setting. If the severity of the breathlessness is low, you can employ self-help measures that include the teaching of breathing exercises. These exercises will focus on implementing slow and deep breathing. Relaxation methods as well as sitting upright in a supportive chair may also positively enhance your airway.

DIZZY SPELLS

Feeling dizzy can be one of the scariest symptoms that someone can present with. This is because it happens so suddenly, with your perception of where you are within your environment causing your body to feel funny. Typically one who has a dizzy spell will feel lightheaded and/or unbalanced. The manner in which this occurs is because the dizzy spells affect the eyes and ears, which is why the end result for some people who have a dizzy spell is fainting. With long COVID-19 having a profound impact on our sensory organs, dizzy spells are common.

With a post-viral illness having the potential to affect all the systems in the human body, when someone has a sudden drop in blood sugar, blood pressure or fluid level, dizzy spells become imminent. However, for such a common symptom, when should you see your doctor? Well, when you feel bouts of dizziness that are accompanied with headaches, a high fever, blurred vision, pins and needles in the extremities, or with a loss in consciousness, an appointment should be made. The treatment of dizziness is based purely on the root cause. For example, simply drinking fluids after intense exercise or heat exposure will relieve the dizziness. In the case of long COVID-19 this can prove difficult, specifically if the person has symptoms that affect many different systems in the human body.

With those that present with constant bouts of dizziness during their long COVID-19 journey, can employ self-help measures. These self-help measures include sitting down immediately when you feel dizzy, using a walker where necessary for the main purpose of improving stability, using handrails on stairs. avoid switching positions suddenly, and stay adequately hydrated by drinking eight glasses of water a day. It is important that caffeine, alcohol and tobacco are avoided as they not only potentiate dizziness episodes, but can also act as a trigger for the dizzy spells to occur.

WEIRD SENSATIONS

Someone who experiences weird sensations can experience a burning, stabbing, itching, crawling and even trickling sensation. With this symptom typically affecting the face first, a person experiencing weird sensations may feel either potentiated or inundated. For example, one may feel severe pain for the simplest of movements like touching a pencil. The contrast then holds true where one does not feel pain when one should, such is the instance if you were to touch a hot stovetop.

People who experience weird sensations as part of long COVID-19 may employ self-help measures which include waiting until the altered sensations spontaneously disappear. However, we want to empower you with physical examples of how to manage your weird sensations. The first step would be to identify any triggers of your weird sensations, and avoiding them where possible. For example, some may be triggered by touch, heat or the feeling of harsh winds on their body–thus avoiding these situations would decrease the chances of you developing weird sensations during your long COVID-19 journey.

Sometimes using a heat pack, cold compress or relaxation technique may aid in the treatment of your weird sensations. However, it all depends on what your triggers are, as this is patient-specific and not a one size fits all approach. Acupuncture and aromatherapy are widely accepted practices that aid in the refocusing of one's bodily sensations. If these modalities aren't effective, one can implement magnetic field treatment to improve the intensity and frequency that you experience your weird sensations.

TINNITUS

Many times we have this ringing in our ears that we have no idea where it came from. Medically, this is what we call tinnitus and it can actually be directly related to an underlying condition. With tinnitus affecting between 15 and 20 percent of people, it may typically be seen with age-related hearing loss. This is when we need to take the patient's profile into account when we look at their long COVID-19. We would need to establish whether the tinnitus is merely due to old age, or whether it is a part of a direct effect from the impact that long COVID-19 has on the human body.

There is a vast array of sounds that you can hear with tinnitus. These include clicking, humming, ringing, buzzing and even roaring. In some cases, the tinnitus can be so loud that it interferes with your ability to concentrate effectively on your tasks. Tinnitus typically resolves itself spontaneously however, if you find that this constant noise either alters pitch, negatively affecting your ability to function, or hinders tasks that you are used to performing, a visit to the doctor is necessary.

It is common that there are specific types of medication that can cause tinnitus, including that of aspiring, some antidepressants and even some antibiotics. It would be important to mention your full medical history to your healthcare professional when speaking to them about your tinnitus. Self-help protocols can be enforced in order to eliminate many of the common causes that would be associated with developing tinnitus. This would be by using hearing protection if you work in a place that is very loud (such as where loud music or machinery are present), turning down the volume when listening to music that is very loud, as well as taking care of your heart health.

Tinnitus is often directly related to a person's heart health thus, by performing regular exercise, eating a healthy and balanced diet, as well as keeping your blood vessels healthy, tinnitus that is associated with your blood vessels can be avoided. It is then optimal that when you visit a healthcare practitioner, you can expect that they may remove earwax build-up, treat a blood vessel condition or even change the medication you are on. Clinically, they may even prescribe that you use a white noise machine, hearing aid, or masking device to decrease the internal load of the tinnitus, making it less bothersome. In some cases an anti-anxiolytic (a medicine that decreases anxiety levels) may even be used, although it may result in drowsiness and nausea being developed.

STOMACH PROBLEMS

With long COVID-19 there is a very high chance of developing some sort of stomach condition, whether it be stomach cramps, diarrhea or a burning sensation that fits snugly within the category of heartburn. When we say someone has a stomach problem, we are referring to any anomaly that causes pain or discomfort. With a post-viral illness, there is a great chance that you will experience stomach problems. Through developing an understanding of long COVID-19, self-help measures should not be discounted, especially where there is evidence of it working.

Visiting a doctor may become a reality when your stomach problems are coupled with blood in the stools or urine, nausea and vomiting that is not handled effectively through self-help means, or whether you lose consciousness during sudden and severe bouts of nausea or pain. However, the silver lining is that there are multiple self-help measures that one can take.

Most causes of stomach problems can be solved through having a healthier diet, better times at which meals are consumed, as well as the consistency of these times. We implore you to utilize the meal planner and nutritional health chart that comes with this book in order to guide you in the right direction. Remember, although medical interventions are effective, they are not always the best option. In the case of stomach problems, natural and holistic therapies have proven to be more efficacious.

EXTREME EMOTIONS

When we look at the alteration of emotions, this can include a difference in its severity, or the movement to the complete opposite scale. For example, an individual could feel more irritable during long COVID-19 than what they typically are, or can go from feeling immensely positive to a feeling of immense depression. It is when we have these intense emotions that we tend to possibly harm relationships with family, friends and fellow coworkers. Emotional dysregulation, especially in the context of long COVID-19 is a complex feeling, primarily because you are isolated because of country restrictions, as well as feeling partially stigmatized at having the coronavirus, along with not being able to have any social interaction to give you a sense of normality.

This form of a finicky situation can be treated in one of two categories. With regards to self-help, if you are able to identify the root cause then you can try to implement measures to curb the intensity of your emotions. For example, if you were an immensely positive person and then developed a severe bout of depression due to lack of social interaction, we know it isn't the same but trying to do some video calls may prove to be beneficial as you are able to keep contact with those that you care about. It is in this manner where mindfulness techniques prove to be useful, primarily because they facilitate the resolution of emotional turmoil by allowing a calm focus towards the root cause. How these mindfulness techniques work, as well as examples of them are discussed a bit later in this book.

With the COVID-19 pandemic causing the shift into virtual consultations it may be a good idea to possibly book a session with a psychologist, just so that you have a completely unbiased approach as well as someone who wants to listen to you and guide you to the right direction. However, we suggest that if the thought crosses your mind to speak with someone else, rather act on that thought than let your emotions build up and erupt all at once.

EBBS AND FLOWS

What we have found very common is that the presentation of someone who has long COVID-19 symbolizes that of a wave. To elaborate this a bit further. It means that there are times where you will feel that you are on the verge of getting better however, the next day could result in you feeling so exhausted and in pain that it feels that you have been hit by a truck. This makes management of long COVID-19 very difficult, especially if you are medication to treat your symptoms. The reason we say this is because many who experience a post-viral illness stop taking their medication as soon as they start to feel better.

This is where the problem comes in, because your body still has traces of the symptom that can magnify and cause a more intense presentation of the symptom later on. Based on the stories that we read in the previous chapter, we see that long COVID-19 can persist for more than 4 months, which poses a large strain on family dynamics, as well as the ability to work and look after your family. With this taken into consideration, following the guidelines in the previous symptom categories can definitely aid in controlling these symptoms effectively, making you feel a little bit more like yourself (which is of great importance).

If you are able to check-in with a healthcare professional, it may set your mind at ease. Joining a long COVID-19 support group may be of great value as you will feel that you are not alone, learn what types of symptoms others are experiencing, as well as learn which nutritional changes and self-help measures to institute. It is learning from the experiences of others that we are able to identify what best works for us. These types of experiences regarding therapies, alternative therapies, how to deal with anxiety, as well as when and how to employ mindfulness techniques into your daily life, will be elaborated on in the coming chapters.

UTTER EXHAUSTION

Have you ever gone to bed rather early, only to sleep more than 10 hours, only to still feel tired (sometimes even more so) when you wake up? This is what most people feel when they are severely exhausted. Exhaustion can be seen as a chronic symptom, especially if the person who has long COVID-19 has previously been diagnosed with depression. Severe exhaustion makes life so much more difficult as needing to explain to others why you don't feel up to anything, and can literally not get out of bed, is a cumbersome task on its own. For many, they find that this too will pass in time however, for others they find that it makes them slip into a downward spiral of negative emotions.

When it comes to self-help measures, research shows that establishing a routine is one of the best ways to overcome severe exhaustion, which to some may seem counterintuitive. It is important that you do not try to do too many things at once. Exhaustion is easier to overcome when you incrementally add a bit more physical exercise each day. Talking to others in a support group as mentioned previously, will definitely aid in being able to find out what works for others and adapt it to suit your own personal needs.

Exhaustion can be overcome, one just needs to find the correct mindset, which may be difficult. However, persistence and trying your utmost best to maintain a positive outlook on your current situation, coupled with the support from your loved ones, will enable you to overcome long COVID-19 successfully.

UNPREDICTABILITY

It is important to realize that the symptoms that you experience during long COVID-19 may intensify and even change. This is why we say that there is a certain element of unpredictability with regards to how the symptoms of your post-viral illness will play out, especially because it is different for each person. Unfortunately, this is why there is no set cure for this unpredictability however, there are means to manage the symptoms that may develop. With the array of developments in alternative treatment modalities, nutritional supplementation and wellbeing practices, long COVID-19 is becoming an illness cured through a holistic approach rather than through purely medical interventions.

Self-help will be directly based on the specific symptom you experience. However, the information above should suffice most of the symptoms that someone will experience as part of long COVID-19. A rule of thumb regarding unpredictability and when to see a doctor, is that as soon as you feel a feeling that you have never felt before a doctor visit should occur, just to lean on the side of caution.

Attention is typically prioritized towards those that are initially affected by the COVID-19 virus, with those experiencing long COVID-19 being kept in the dark. With over 10% of individuals experiencing the virus for periods longer than three weeks, there is a greater need for long COVID-19 to be acknowledged as a complication of COVID-19. With long COVID-19 resulting in patients being too ill to work, whilst experiencing relapsing symptoms, it is important that long COVID-19 gets the attention that it deserves. This is why it is important to implement self-help measures within your recovery process, as it focuses on your own body's defense mechanism rather than what medicines can do for you. With individuals who deal with long-COVID-19 regularly resorting to social media for help regarding their symptoms, we felt that describing the most common long COVID-19 symptoms, as well as shifting their mindset towards the self-help options that are available, would be of great benefit for those fighting a post-viral illness.

CHAPTER 4

LONG-TERM EFFECTS

"The results are very surprising. These results suggest that players may be playing [despite] injuries to their long-term detriment."
–Michael Collins

L ong COVID-19 is typically seen as having long-term effects. This is in essence why we call it 'long' COVID-19. However, what we need to be wary of is that the length of long COVID-19 is not definitive. Some people will experience long COVID-19 for one month, and others for four months. This is why it is of utmost importance that you remain wary of any developing symptoms so that you can combat them as quickly as possible, which will ensure a minimal effect on your daily functioning. You've already had COVID-19, we want to make sure that you do not have to put your life on hold any longer.

With the definition of a long-term illness being one that is present for at least six months, long COVID-19 truly has the potential to fit this definition With the incidence of long COVID-19 being on the rise, especially as infections skyrocket worldwide, with modern-day treatments and educating of patients, one does not need to feel captivated by their illness. What we have discovered is that it is very difficult to find good medical advice, whether it be directly related to your illness or contrastingly about living a more balanced and healthier lifestyle. This is where we come in. We will discuss what you can do (or even that of your friends or family) in order to ensure that you maintain the best quality of life that you possibly can whilst traversing through long COVID-19.

It is important that when looking at the long-term effects of long COVID-19, that you find reliable information regarding the condition, as this gives you the autonomy to really have control over the illness. If you are taking any form of medication to help curb the long COVID-19 symptoms, make sure that you have consulted a health-care practitioner or pharmacist regarding any special instructions, storage conditions, as well as doses and potential side effects that could arise.

What one can typically expect with long COVID-19 is what can feel like a constant battle with being able to regain a sense of normality. We are not going to create a delusion that it is going to be an easy journey. However, what we want to do is give you the best possible chance in order to fight back against this illness. What we would highly recommend is trying to explain to those that you interact with on a daily basis what you are going through. It may be difficult for them to understand because they themselves are not going through long COVID-19. It is when you establish this open communication that you do not have to feel ashamed of how you are feeling.

When we look specifically at long COVID-19 the most common signs that tend to linger over time will include fatigue, having a cough coupled with being short of breath, constant and persistent headaches, and joint pain. What you want to ensure is that you make regular check-ups with your healthcare professional in order to ensure that the lingering symptoms that progress throughout long COVID-19 are not due to any underlying conditions. We say this because during your initial COVID-19 infection, depending on the severity, your heart, lungs or brain may have been compromised. This is why it is so important to ensure that you are always open and honest with your healthcare professionals regarding how you are feeling so that they can provide the best care possible for you. We want to equip you with some key steps in order to ensure that you are able to manage your long COVID-19 effects adequately, whilst ensuring there is no further development of other symptoms.

The first step is to ensure that you eat healthy foods and do not neglect your nutritional requirements. We tend to forget that once one gets sick, it is the presence of specific vitamins and minerals that enable us to feel better faster. For example, when we either harm our skin or feel that our bones are weak, vitamin A supplementation can be taken to enhance their time for repair. We then have vitamin C that is important in the formation of collagen, a protein of our connective tissue. So, when we couple our nutritional requirements with that of the medicines provided by our healthcare professional, our care becomes optimized. It is when people are healthy that they tend to steer clear from bad dietary habits that impede the healing process. You may feel that coffee is a pick-me-up however, when you are ill it prolongs your illness journey, making recovery that much harder to achieve.

So you see, it is only once we are well informed that we can start making strategic decisions in being able to combat long COVID-19 effectively. Moving into an example of nutritional proportions, it is recommended that you eat five times a day. Now, this doesn't mean wolfing down absolutely everything your eyes land on. What it means is that you eat three small to medium meals a day along with two nutritious snacks. What this ensures so that you do not have any drops in your blood sugar that result in you feeling fatigued.

It is important that you feed your body with carbohydrates that have a low glycemic index. What this ensures is that there are not sudden blood sugar spikes and that there is no potential spike in inflammation throughout your body. With the intake of proteins giving you the energy to go about your daily activities, whilst rebuilding the cells in your body, it is generally advised to get about 15 to 20 percent of your calories from protein. Plant-based proteins tend to have advantages over animal proteins as phytochemicals within the plant-based proteins ensure that your body reestablishes its sense of equilibrium from before you were infected with COVID-19. Fruits and vegetables are key in providing your body with the vitamins and minerals needed to heal itself. As a general rule, darker colored fruits and vegetables are rich in phytochemicals and antioxidants than that of light-colored ones. This is why it is important to eat at least five servings of fruits and vegetables each day. When visiting your healthcare professional, you may be advised to obtain a supplement that gives your body a boost in fighting the symptoms of long

COVID-19. Many would recommend a multivitamin, primarily because it is very rare that you will be able to obtain all the vitamins and minerals necessary for your body, in their required amounts, every single day.

The second step is to ensure that you get enough sleep. With long COVID-19 making you feel drained and not in the mood to do anything, one needs to give your body ample time to recover. You may find that your healthcare professional may even give you some melatonin (which is naturally produced by our body's pineal gland) in order to not only help in the regulation of your sleep cycle, but also to help repair any form of corrupt DNA that may have been present as a result of either the initial COVID-19 infection, or as a part of the post-viral illness.

What tends to elevate stress levels in individuals who have long COVID-19, is that you are missing sleep based on discomfort and possible anxiety spikes. The last thing that you need is for these sleepless nights to harm your recovery rate. What is of importance is that you start to document how much sleep you get, as well as what you find to be interfering with it. You can either do this by making a sleep journal, or by using wearable technology to track your sleep cycles more effectively. You will then be able to identify the regular causes of your sleep disturbances which would range from pain to anxiety and even needing to go to the bathroom. It is in this way that you are empowered to identify your main causes, and tackle them one by one.

The third step in being able to manage the long-term effects of long

COVID-19 is by ensuring that you get out of bed and get your heart pumping. For many they may think there is an inconsistency with needing to rest but then also needing to get their bodies to move around. Exercise is seen as being highly beneficial in regulating the balancing in our bodies in terms of intrinsic functioning. This means that all of the chemicals in our body are kept functioning like a well-oiled machine. Exercise produces some of these chemicals, ensuring that we are not only feeling better and have a quicker recovery rate, but also allows for the strengthening of muscles, tendons, ligaments and bones that may have been weakened from not being as active as before needing to deal with a post-viral illness.

The proof is in the pudding, and this is shown by a study that was conducted by Ohio State University in 2005 whereby individuals were given a small wound. Half of the participants were put into an aerobic exercise program, whilst the other half were told to go about their daily lives and consciously not make an effort to perform any specific exercises. It took exercisers a total of 29 days for the wound to heal, compared to 39 days for nonexercisers.

Now at this point you may ask how you are expected to do exercise when one of the most common symptoms of long COVID-19 is joint pain. Lucky for you this exact concept has been studied in depth where they say that you can perform non-weight-bearing exercises that get your blood pumping. These types of exercises include swimming, as well as performing isometric exercises which have the main focus on relaxing and contracting your muscles. Leg lifts can also be performed as there is no direct force that is acting on and stressing your joints.

It is important to realize that having an illness, whether it be post-viral or something else down the line, it is an unavoidable part of life. However, our bodies want to heal, they want to overcome any obstacles that present themselves. With long COVID-19 there is no need to accept a "new normal" too soon. Through being able to put your mind to it whilst following the ideas we have listed in this chapter, your body and your mind will be able to help fight against this illness. It is important to ensure that you employ mental strategies to boost your body's potential to heal effectively. Focus on reducing any pain that you may feel.

Acknowledging the relationship between your mind and your body will ensure that you do not further weaken your immune system. What we mean by this is biological in nature. By decreasing stress levels you are ultimately increasing the ability of your body to fight against the symptoms that are associated with long COVID-19. By being able to effectively monitor your mood, surround yourselves with those that you love, as well as remaining grounded in your spirituality, your long-term effects will ameliorate much quicker and you will be back to living your life before COVID-19 quicker than you ever imagined.

2

Practical Steps Towards Coping With Long COVID-19

Contents:

CHAPTER 5

SELF-HELP

"I cannot do all the good that the world needs. But the world needs all the
good that I can do"
—Jana Stanfield

S elf-help is a key factor in being able to effectively overcome
long COVID-19. As we have learned with long COVID-19,
there is no specific timeline for recovery. Depending on how
well you listen to your body, follow the directions as stipulated above,
as well as take the medications as prescribed by your healthcare professional, you will cut your recovery time dramatically. However, in
order to give you some timeframe regarding how long recovery can
take, it can be anywhere between three weeks to seven months after
having been infected with COVID-19.

What we want to ensure is that we are able to provide you with
measures that allow you to be realistic regarding your recovery with
long COVID-19. What we do not want, is to give you information
that promises to work in 1 week, only for that to not be the case and

you start feeling heightened feelings of depression and anxiety. This is bound to negatively affect your recovery rate, as well as remove any inclination that you may have had to fight this long COVID-19 illness head-on.

It is important that we learn to take time out in order to avoid any further complications of long COVID-19. What this means is that when we are not feeling our best, we should not purposefully place ourselves in situations that require us to overexert our already compromised states. If your main job was looking after the kids, then ask your significant other to look after them while you rest up. If need be, call in the cavalry, whether it be close friends or family in order to assist you on your road to recovery. The worst thing you can do is allow your pride to come in between your ability to recover as quickly as possible. In this time focus on you and your health. If you aren't up to checking work emails, or even from working from home, then do not hinder your recovery by not switching off properly.

We have seen how quickly viruses can spread, and it is for this reason why one needs to remain certain that they are out of the woods before even attempting unnecessary contact with the outside world. It is important to be realistic with yourself. If the self-help techniques that you have employed within your recovery plan are not working effectively or as quickly as you hoped it would, it is time to visit your local healthcare facility for a thorough check-up. Now is not the time to be a hero, it is the time that you need to rest and recover so that you can be the hero to others.

One needs to be realistic with their capabilities as they progress towards recovering completely. Especially if your long COVID-19 symptoms have lasted for a rather long period (e.g., four months), you cannot expect your body to be fully operational within 24 hours of not feeling nauseous anymore. You need to be able to be disciplined enough that you set realistic goals with how you integrate yourself back into society once you have fully recovered. When a professional athlete could swim 150 laps of the pool at their peak form, they need to be realistic and acknowledge that they won't be able to go near that number within the next few weeks and months that follow, finally recovering from a post-viral illness.

When you are going through a post-viral illness you need to ensure that you look after your gut. This specific aspect was discussed in previous chapters, however, we are going to give you a bit of a deeper understanding of what actually goes on in your body. With self-help techniques that focus on your gut, you want to take into consideration the importance of having healthy gut bacteria in your gut. This becomes even more important when you have gut-related symptoms as part of your long COVID-19 journey. This is because episodes of diarrhea tend to affect the guts microbiome, throwing it out of balance. What you can definitely do as a part of your self-help plan, is to actively replenish these gut bacteria by implementing the use of probiotics into your recovery regime. Typically one should look at probiotics that contain Bifidobacterium and lactobacillus as these are the most researched strains. It is also important that when you take your probiotics, that you do not take it with hot water as it will decrease the number of bacteria that will reach the gut.

It is difficult to know exactly what to eat when you are going through an illness, especially one as complex as long COVID-19. This is why it is important to retrain your appetite. By this we mean that you can start introducing foods into your body at a slow pace. If you are used to eating the recommended five meals as we mentioned previously, and have only had the appetite of one piece of toast throughout your illness journey, then it is definitely not a good idea to jump straight back to five meals. The reason we say this is because our bodies adapt to being ill and to the amount of food we consume. By overloading the body too quickly, the body will go into a form of nutrient shock that will hinder the absorbance of these vitamins and minerals. This will also result in you feeling very ill, over and above how you are feeling due to long COVID-19.

Ensuring that you are drinking enough fluids throughout your illness journey is of vital importance. Especially with a post-viral illness, our bodies rely heavily on adequate hydration in order for our immune systems to be able to function effectively. However, this does not mean that you can ingest alcohol, coffee and milkshakes. Alcohol, as well as dairy-rich drinks, have a negative impact on the functioning of your immune system. This is why it is recommended that you focus more on drinking water, juice from juiced fruits, and herbal teas. Remaining hydrated is even more important when you start to introduce exercise into your daily life again. If you jump into your normal routine whilst not remaining hydrated, there is a high chance that your blood sugar will drop too fast and you will end up losing consciousness.

Allow yourself to be a beginner again, even if it only temporarily. As someone who does not know when the end of their long COVID-19 journey will come, you need to remain cognizant of your body's capabilities when you start to feel better. Many have found that adopting a personalized wellbeing plan has aided their self-help journey through long COVID-19, as well as facilitating their bodies in being able to reach its previous potential and activity level. With a personalized wellbeing plan, you are able to share what matters to you, as well as effectively communicate how people can best support you through your journey. It is also seen as a form of reflection where it provides a quick summary of what matters to you, primarily so that you do not have to explain the same story to everyone that asks.

The contents of a personalized wellbeing plan are adapted to the person progressing through long COVID-19. This means that there will be general information about the ill person, focusing on details that may be necessary for a carer or family member when they come over to check-in on you. There will also be information about your health history, any previous illnesses, as well as the medications that you are taking. It is important that when listing all your medication, you include herbal supplements, current medication that you are using to manage your long COVID-19 symptoms, as well as any medication that you are taking to treat another chronic disease. This will give a great overview of any visiting healthcare professional regarding your current state of health, as well as where alterations can be made to maximize your quality of life and rate of recovery.

The introspection portion of the personalized wellbeing plan allows you to think of what really matters right now. The types of questions you can think about include:

- Who are the people that I consider to be the most important in my life?

- What are the normal means of communication that I use in order to stay in touch with them?

- How will I need to alter my communication strategies in order to keep in touch with them now, especially in the time of this pandemic?

- What are the routines that I find important in my life?

- What do I miss doing which I could do before?

The importance of these questions is to ensure that the decreased energy that you do have is spent in the most concise manner, on what truly matters. When one employs self-help strategies, it isn't merely just to focus on your physical health, but also your mental health. Your mental health is of immense importance, especially in times of self-isolation. This is why employing self-help strategies that impact you on a holistic level is the best approach that you can take.

CHAPTER 6

TREATMENTS

"The more perfect a thing is, the more susceptible to good and bad treatment it is."
–Dante Alighieri

Treatments for long COVID-19 are typically directly based on the symptoms that each person experiences, as well as the severity of these symptoms. However, there is one very specific syndrome that long COVID-19 patients experience, and that is post-viral fatigue syndrome. It is because of the difficulty associated with diagnosing this syndrome, primarily because fatigue is a core symptom of long COVID-19, that is often overlooked when working up a patient.

This means that post-viral fatigue will only be diagnosed once all other causes of your fatigue have been tested and ruled out. What is highly recommended during your long COVID-19 journey is that you analyze all of your symptoms individually, focussing on how fatigued they make you feel. This becomes vital information when you are visiting your healthcare professional for a check-in. What you can add here is whether you are experiencing any other mental health symptoms such as depression or anxiety. The reason these symptoms are of importance as they themselves can present with severe levels of fatigue and if not noted, may mimic post-viral fatigue syndrome. The healthcare professional may also request a blood test to rule out other medical-related causes of fatigue which include diabetes, anemia or hypothyroidism (which is when your thyroid gland is not producing the correct amounts of chemicals needed for your body to function optimally). An exercise-stress test may also be done to rule out any heart or lung conditions, as well as a sleep study that will rule out sleep disorders (e.g., insomnia) that are affecting your quality of sleep, leaving you constantly fatigued.

Now the real question arises, how does one go about treating post-viral fatigue? Seeing as there is still no concrete evidence that lets us know why post-viral fatigue happens, the treatment is solely based on the management of your symptoms. This is why management includes taking over-the-counter pain relievers that are able to relieve any lingering pain that is hindering your ability to obtain good quality sleep. When one is fatigued, there is a sort of fuzziness to our thoughts, where we cannot seem to concentrate or remember tasks that need to be done. A manner to overcome this is by using a calendar or organizer to help with these memory and concentration issues. It is in this way that you can also rank the necessity of these tasks, seeing as whilst you are recovering from long COVID-19 it is important that you do not overexert yourself.

One of the other ways of dealing with post-viral fatigue is by delegating daily activities where possible to conserve energy, whilst focusin on relaxation techniques to ground your thoughts and emotions. It is noted that post-viral fatigue can pose to be highly frustrating, and even more so seeing as you have already had your body fight through the initial viral infection. However, the good news is that the aid listed is bound to help at least 90% of patients that present with post-viral fatigue syndrome. The other 10% have looked for resources elsewhere, reaching out to support groups to see if there are any unconventional methods that will work for them.

Now although it is important to remind yourself that your symptoms during long COVID-19 may change, it is not at all an indication of how long your recovery will take. This is why the best you can do is ensure that you are treating your symptoms effectively. With having a fever being a common occurrence both through COVID-19's initial infection as well as through long COVID-19, there are definitely some non-medical and medical treatment regimens that can be performed.

Non-medical treatment modalities include ensuring that you always remain hydrated, as when you have a fever the chances of you becoming dehydrated increase greatly. The manner in which you become dehydrated is when the evaporation of moisture from your skin occurs primarily due to the body trying to cool itself off by sweating. If you find that the room that you are mostly in is immensely warm, it is a good idea to cool it down by opening up windows and allowing adequate ventilation to circulate throughout the room. It is important to note that placing a cold compress on someone's head when they have a fever is not recommended. This is because the blood vessels will constrict if the water is too cold, resulting in a reduction in the amount of heat that is being lost by the body, thus trapping heat in the deeper parts of the body.

Having a cough is another very common symptom that may be associated with your long COVID-19 journey. However, the treatment here will depend on the type of cough that you have. Here we will look at both a dry cough and a wet cough. With a dry cough, the act of coughing occurs more frequently, as well as when one is laying flat on their back. This means that there is potential for sleep to be hindered when having a cough. Treatment for a dry cough may include a cough suppressant, and pain medication if there are aches and pains associated. However, it is important to note that with a wet cough, there may be an underlying bacterial infection present that would prompt the use of antibiotics. Antibiotics are not to be given for viral infections. Treating coughs due to viral infections can include inhaling steam to moisten your dried mucous membranes, as well as using honey and lemon drops to aid in the soothing of your throat.

Shortness of breath is a symptom that 90% of patients with long COVID-19 experience. With this symptom, it is important that if you are a smoker that you stop immediately as it will definitely contribute negatively towards your breathing quality, as well as the development of a dry cough. There are both medical and nonmedical manners to overcome shortness of breath. Looking at the medical alternatives, they are primarily focused on the causative agent. This means that if you are struggling to breathe after doing a large amount of exercise or physical work while you are sick, you will most likely be given an inhaler that relieves any constriction in your airways, thus promoting good airflow. If you are one that already had an underlying respiratory condition prior to long COVID-19, it may be required to increase the dose of your corticosteroid inhaler. People who have these severe bouts of breathlessness due to long COVID-19, can also be put on a short course of an oral corticosteroid (e.g., prednisone) in order to aid in removing any intrinsic inflammation of the airways.

In terms of nonmedical treatment modalities, breathlessness can be tackled by ensuring you do not perform too many physically demanding tasks in one go. This correlates with the previous chapter and how you need to ensure that you are easing yourself back into your physical fitness regimen rather than believing that you are in your same form before you were infected with COVID-19. Shortness of breath can also be aided by losing weight if you are overweight, sleeping with your head slightly raised on more pillows, as well as performing non-weight-bearing exercises that include yoga.

Looking at headaches, treatment is directed at the type of headache that is experienced. It is based on the severity and longevity of the headache in question. With adequate meditation practices, stress-induced migraines and cluster headaches can be prevented. This is primarily because meditation targets the areas of the nervous system that focus on stress, deterring the physical manifestations of stress away from the feeling thereof. Acupuncture has also proved useful as the needles are placed along the neck and at the base of the head. How acupuncture is effective is by blocking the movement of pain to your nervous system, interrupting the message and alleviating your pain. Localized massage therapy is typically used along with acupuncture and cognitive brain therapy in order to provide long-term relief of one's headaches.

Migraines that are associated with long COVID-19 present with intense pain that pulsates, adding an associated amount of nausea, vomiting and an increased sensitivity to external stimuli. Typically, the only form of non-medical treatment that is warranted with migraines, is to rest in a quiet and dark room, along with very small amounts of caffeine. Medical management includes the over-the-counter pain medications as is that for tension-type headaches. However, due to the severity of the headache, it would be necessary to be placed on prescription medication after consultation with your healthcare professional. These types of medications are known as the triptans, and include sumatriptan and zolmitriptan. For those that find they are getting migraines frequently during long COVID-19, preventative medications may be the most appropriate choice. Examples of some of these medications include propranolol, topiramate and metoprolol.

Headaches can definitely hinder your everyday functioning, but in most cases it is nothing to worry about. However, if you find that the headaches that you get are interrupting your personal life, it is recommended to visit your local healthcare facility for an adequate work-up to be performed. In the case of long COVID-19, headaches cannot always be prevented, but it definitely can be treated.

It is these treatment modalities that are supported and instituted by world-renowned healthcare organizations. These organizations include the National Health Services (NHS) as well as the World Health Organization (WHO). It is important to remember that these modalities are not a cure for long COVID-19, but are measures that can be instituted in order to increase your quality of life, as well as decrease your physical symptoms whilst you progress through your long COVID-19 journey.

CHAPTER 7

THERAPY

"Smile, it's free therapy"
—Doug Horton

Seeing as post-viral illnesses have not been actively discussed and investigated as it should've been, that does not necessarily mean that there is no information on it. With post-viral syndrome, the fun fact is that it can even develop after a simple bout of flu or infection with the common cold. With the core cause of post-viral illness being unknown, it has been discovered that it is the manner in which our body reacts to the virus upon initial presentation, which will dictate whether we experience a post-viral illness or not. Some medical professionals have dedicated years of their life to studying post-viral illness, and are starting to attribute it to possible inflammation in the brain. It is the immune response that our body has towards the post-viral illness that causes us to experience symptoms.

Apart from COVID-19, there are a variety of other forms of viruses that, when infecting the human body, can trigger a post-viral syndrome. Examples of these include pneumonia, the common cold, flu, herpes and HIV. For some, especially for those that are on medication or suffer from conditions that weaken their immune systems, post-viral illness symptoms in itself will be more common. With the symptoms varying from person to person, there is a typical presentation for individuals that have long COVID-19. These individuals will describe themselves as feeling severely fatigued as well as generally unwell. The trick that will allow you to diagnose a post-viral illness is that these symptoms remain, irrespective of how many hours the person sleeps, or how well they take care of themselves.

It is in this way that the post-viral syndrome causes additional symptoms that are unrelated to long COVID-19. These symptoms range from confusion to having swollen lymph nodes. Seeing as the medical community has different views and perspectives of what constitutes long COVID-19, the recommendations may differ slightly. However, in most cases, treating the symptoms until the person feels closer to the end of the road to recovery, tends to be the best option. Although there has been much talk and interest regarding which over-the-counter medications to give, the most common medical treatment regimens were discussed in the previous chapter.

Taking a look at some home remedies, many of them have a lifestyle component to them. The main reason one would focus on lifestyle alterations is that the support of the human body then occurs. This support comes from the nutrients and minerals within the diet, sleeping seven to nine hours each night, implementing mindfulness practices, ensuring that you maintain adequately hydrated, and that you avoid foods that are laden with grease.

THE 3 PS

Much of the therapy that is associated with long COVID-19 focuses on conserving energy. However, what is coming to light as the COVID-19 pandemic progresses, is that rehabilitation needs to be seen as the number one priority. It is when you are ill that you feel tired and do not have much energy to expend. You know you have reached this state when the simplest of everyday tasks feel like hard work. These tasks can be anything from putting on your shoes, to taking a plate to the kitchen. In order to focus on conserving your energy, the 3 Ps principle was created by the Royal College of Occupational Therapists. These Ps focus on pace, plan and prioritizing.

PACE

It is important to learn to pace your activities, especially when you are recovering from a post-viral illness. It is through pacing yourself that you will be able to have enough energy in order to ensure that you can effectively complete an activity. It is scientifically proven that individuals will recover faster if they decide to work on a task until they are tired, in contrast to when they are exhausted. Terming the exhaustion "the big push" is what will leave you feeling as if you are in a constant vegetative state, with absolutely zero energy, as well as a longer recovery time.

In order to provide some context to the pacing approach, we will use the following example. If someone were to use the big push approach, they would climb all the stairs of a building all in one go, resulting in them needing to rest for 10 minutes as soon as they reach the top. This will also result in them feeling aches and pains the next day, primarily due to the overexertion of their muscles. When we take the same scenario and place it into the pacing approach, what we find is that by climbing five steps at a time with 30-second intervals will result in you needing a shorter rest at the top, as well as not feeling as physically taxed the next day.

Some tips to ensure that when pacing, you conserve as much energy as possible, is by breaking up activities into smaller tasks that you can perform throughout the day. Many find that building rest times into their schedules make them feel more energized, as well as allow you to be more productive. The recommended resting time that should be allocated after completing a segment of a task is 30-40 minutes. When in doubt, take a seat and have a bit of a rest.

PLAN

What we want to do at this stage is take some time to critically analyze the activities that you are used to doing during a day and the given week. Long COVID-19 will drastically affect your ability to perform these tasks. This is why it is important to prioritize and reevaluate the tasks that you are used to doing. You can ask yourself questions to help you make these choices. An example can include, "Do I need to do this task this week? Is it possible that I can perform this task every two weeks?"

It is important that we also think of the times that an activity will typically take place. If you find that you are busier in the morning, then rather schedule your bath and shower time for the evenings when you can relax. Spread out your must-do tasks across the week. If you know that you need to do laundry, fix up the garden, as well as go to the supermarket for food, space them out across the week in order to ensure that you have enough time to rest in order to replenish your energy levels before tackling the next task.

Here some tips that we have is to collect all the items that you need before a task. It is in this way that you do not spend any unnecessary time and energy on locating everything whilst doing the task. Do not be shy to ask family or friends for assistance, as this will most likely allow you to get that much more done throughout the day.

PRIORITIZE

Prioritizing tasks works hand-in-hand with planning these tasks as you start to identify which tasks are important and require a space in your week. It is here that we want to invite you to perform some more introspection about where you are in terms of your long COVID-19 recovery journey. Some of the questions that you can ask are the following:

- What tasks are of absolute necessity to get done today?

- Are there any tasks that I would like to do today, given that I have the time and the energy to do them?

- What tasks are there that do not need to be done immediately, and that I can push to a later day or week?

• Are there tasks that someone else can help me with or do for me?

The rule of thumb when it comes to conserving energy, is that you want to avoid any bodily functions that will require extra effort. This means that you should steer clear from, or ask for someone's aid with tasks that include either reaching, bending, lifting or twisting. In terms of body positioning, especially when we want to pick up an item, research shows that by bending with your knees, you are expending less energy than if you were to bend from your waist.

Throughout this chapter we have seen alternative manners and methods that are available for the treatment of long COVID-19. Many of these therapies focus on not only aiding in the treatment of long COVID-19, but also on enhancing the management of the related symptoms. Although there are many symptoms that long COVID-19 can present with, there are manners which include planning your day and prioritizing your tasks, which will decrease the anxiety levels felt throughout the day, tackling more than one symptom by adjusting one to two aspects of your life.

CHAPTER 8

ALTERNATIVE THERAPY

"Men and nations behave wisely once they have exhausted all the other alternatives."

–Abba Eban

L et's take a minute and shift our focus to treatments that would fall out of the mainstream concept of healthcare. By this, we want to refer to how complementary and alternative medicines are able to act as treatment modalities for long COVID-19. These types of medicines and treatments will typically range from using homeopathy, to aromatherapy, and even including meditation, acupuncture and colonic irrigation.

Many first hear about complementary medicine and treatment modalities from the support groups that they have found online. Knowing that there is someone that is also on a long COVID-19 recovery journey finding success in effectively treating their symptoms, gives one the hope needed to take the next step and make an appointment with a healthcare professional that specializes in alternative medicine practices. This is the prime manner in which the symptoms of long COVID-19 can be treated effectively.

What is important to note about the use of complementary and alternative medicines is that there are varying levels of evidence depending on what treatment modalities are seen as being safe and effective. Luckily for us, there is an index that contains a list of all the conditions and their complementary and alternative treatments on the NHS website. Delving a bit deeper into how these alternative treatment modalities are used, many of them have proved to be effective when treating the symptoms associated with long COVID-19.

Acupuncture is seen as being a fantastic substitute to relieving pain and headache in those that despise taking any form of oral medicine. With acupuncture, the practice involved inserting very fine needles into different parts of your body. These parts, termed acupuncture points, are distinct areas that have been trialed and repeated to show the alleviation of specific symptoms and areas where the symptom usually occurs. For example, one of the acupuncture points for a headache lies in the groove of the muscles on either side of the spine, in the neck region.

The use of acupuncture is based on the belief that one's energy has been blocked, with this blockage being the primary reason for your health problems. Through acupuncture you are able to unblock your energy channels in a way that restores energy flow, thus alleviating the health problems. With the use of acupuncture being primarily for headaches or chronic pain, promising research is being established with its use in aiding the relief of depression and anxiety. The British Medical Acupuncture Society, as well as that of The British Acupuncture Council provides stellar information regarding the research obtained for the efficacy of acupuncture in being able to relieve headaches, chronic pain, anxiety and depression.

Aromatherapy has gotten much international exposure, especially as the use of essential oils has shown researched efficacy in having healing properties. Many find that the smell of the essential oils promotes heightened relaxation, allowing them to obtain a better quality of sleep. Research has also shown that there are smells that are used to relieve pain and improve a depressed mood. Aromatherapy has been used largely within the long COVID-19 context as the symptoms that essential oils can treat directly relate to the symptoms that people with long COVID-19 experience. An example of this is using lavender and camomile essential oils to aid your relaxing, clear mind fog, promote better quality sleep and alleviate light headaches.

The diversity that exists with using essential oils is astounding. Essential oils can be incorporated into creams, used in oil burners, massaged directly into the skin, and even added into a warm bath. However, no modality is without fault as there is a chance that you can develop an allergic reaction to some essential oils. This is why it is of utmost importance to make an appointment with an aromatherapist before using essential oils, or by contacting your country's aromatherapy council for more information.

The Bowen technique is a rather new form of complementary medicine, which focuses on light touches on a person's skin, in a manner that uses gentle rolling motions. With this form of contact therapy, there has been much research done, showing that the use of this technique is used for physical problems. The range of these physical problems is currently what is being studied in more depth however, the progress in terms of decreasing levels of depression, anxiety and stress, has been proven. The Bowen Therapy Professionals Association contains up-to-date information that will result in answering any of the questions you may have about this technique.

One of the most common forms of alternative medicine in being able to treat long COVID-19 symptoms is homeopathy. Homeopathy involves the use of diluted natural substances in order to treat both physical and mental health care problems. What we find with homeopaths is that they believe that the more a substance can be diluted, the more effective it will be. However, there are large levels of controversy regarding whether homeopathy actually works. Despite the ongoing conflict between science-based and natural products based healthcare professionals, there are those that have used homeopathic remedies successfully, stating that it did indeed help in relieving their stress, depression, tinnitus and anxiety levels, whilst suppressing the pain associated with headaches.

Looking at the more mental effects that long COVID-19 has on a person, meditation has shown to be of some benefit. It is when you are able to quieten your mind and calm your mind, that you are able to rest and relax your mind, calming your nerves and diminishing your anxiety levels. What is great about meditation is that it can incorporate degrees of mindfulness, allowing you to focus on your own wellbeing as you continue through your long COVID-19 journey. It is in this day and age that we thank the internet, primarily for the apps and free online videos that teach us how to meditate effectively, whilst being mindful and managing our negative emotions and feelings of stress.

A fantastic form of complementary and alternative treatment is reflexology. With reflexology being slightly related to acupressure and acupuncture, where it is different is that it focuses solely on your feet, hands, ears and face. The belief in reflexology is that there are nerves of the nervous system that are linked to organs in our body from our extremities and face. It is this way that many have experienced positive results when visiting a reflexologist for their aid in eliminating symptoms associated with long COVID-19. Participants in long COVID-19 support groups have expressed their surprise that reflexology was able to remove their stomach problems, as well as lift their self-esteem and self-confidence, ameliorating any feelings of anxiety and self-doubt that presented itself.

Many people who suffer from long COVID-19 may feel that they prefer the approach of spiritual and energy healing. When referring to this form of complementary treatment, it is believed that one has both a physical and an energy body. With many spiritual and energy healers believing that the healthier your energy body the greater the positive impact on your mental health. The primary manner in which the rectification of one's energy body is done is performing Reiki, a traditional form of Japanese healing therapy. Although there is not much research that has been done into the effects of energy healing on one's mental health, there are success stories of individuals who possessed a post-viral illness, feeling less depressed and stress free.

A form of alternative therapy that is growing in popularity regarding the treatment of post-viral illness symptoms, is that of osteopathy and chiropractic. Classified as manipulation therapies, the practitioner will use their hands to work on your joints, ligaments, tendons, muscles and tissues. Typically, these forms of alternative therapy are used to treat pain that is associated with the lower back, neck and shoulder however, there has also been proof that it can assist in the management of sport injuries and recurrent headaches. Some individuals get rather freaked out when these practitioners use spinal manipulation, focussing on moving your joints through a specific range of motion, ending with a high-speed thrust that makes a large cracking sound as your joints return to their correct positions.

Accessing and utilizing complementary therapies is a mixed and rather uncertain field. The reason for this is that there is not as much research as one would find with conventional therapies. However, in terms of the National Institute for Health and Care Excellence, there are large amounts of research being done to create a comparative approach between alternative medicine and conventional medicines.

Many research results have actually shown a favorable result for complementary therapies over that of conventional therapies. However, if you find that using complementary medicine, especially to manage your long COVID-19 symptoms, works for you, then we suggest you continue using it. What many have employed is combining complementary medicine with mindfulness practices in order to enhance the positive attitude that they have towards their choice of therapy.

One of the main goals of treating long COVID-19 is the alleviation of symptoms. It doesn't matter whether this is obtained via conventional or complementary means, if your symptoms are alleviated, you are on the road to a speedy and less treacherous recovery.

CHAPTER 9

NUTRITION AND SUPPLEMENTS

"We are all warned to read labels. The salutary truth is that we shouldn't be eating anything that has a label on it!"
—T.C. Fry

A dequate nutrition and supplementation are imperative in speeding up the recovery rate that your body has towards long COVID-19 and any other post-viral illness. However, there are so many claims that specific foods and supplements will unrealistically make you feel better faster than what one would believe to be realistically possible. This is why we want to tailor this information regarding nutrition and supplementation that can be used, which should be omitted as well as which foods you should focus on consuming during your recovery journey.

We previously discussed the implementation of probiotics in order to reinstate the balance of the good bacteria that are present in the gut. This is especially useful based on the symptom profile of long COVID-19, where gut and stomach problems remain a common occurrence. Delving deeper into the biology of the gut bacteria, up to 80% of the immune cells that give our body's our immunity, are located in the gut. Thus, if there is a direct impact in the gut, our body's immunity will plummet. This is why we need to focus on replenishing our gut's good bacteria, especially when dealing with long COVID-19. Natural yogurts and probiotic drinks are where these good bacteria are mostly found. Further examples of this good bacteria include that of *L. bulgaricus*, *L. casei* and *S. thermophilus*.

Taking a closer look at the constituents of foodstuffs, it is emphasized that those who have long COVID-19 focus on the amount of protein that is ingested. Our bodies use protein to repair damaged tissues as well as build and strengthen the micro-environment of these internal tissues. Furthermore, proteins act as building blocks for important enzymes, hormones, skin tissue, muscle, cartilage and blood. Thus, seeing as protein is such an important molecule, the Harvard School of Public Health recommends that 46 to 56 grams of protein be ingested every day. Up to 65 grams may be recommended, especially for those that are currently diagnosed with a post-viral illness. The type of foods that you would look at in order to obtain your protein would be your lean meats, nuts and seeds, fish, beans poultry, tofu and spinach. It is important to also take in sufficient amounts of fats and carbohydrates as recommended by your dietitian or healthcare professional. The reason for this is that it ensures that your ingested proteins are not used as an energy source, but as an adjunct to healing damaged tissue.

Focussing on foods that have high levels of vitamin C in them will definitely positively influence your body. The role of vitamin C in the body is that it not only increases the absorption of iron, but also acts as an antioxidant to help your cells recover from fighting your post-viral illness. With long COVID-19 still resulting in possible traces of the initial COVID-19 infection, ingesting vitamin C will aid in the body's stimulation of white blood cells, contributing to the attacking and destruction of infectious pathogens. It is important to note that vitamin C is classified as a water-soluble vitamin. What this means is that one needs to regularly ingest food sources that have this vitamin on a daily basis as there are no designated areas of storage for it in the human body. Foods that have a high level of vitamin C include strawberries, kiwis, papayas and bell peppers.

Other vitamins that also need to be taken include vitamin A and B. With vitamin A, there is support in the maintenance of healthy teeth, including that of soft tissue, the skin, as well as its associated mucus membranes. Vitamin A further plays a vital role in keeping our eyes healthy by balancing the necessary pigments that are present. With the effects of long COVID-19 possibly affecting one's quality of vision as a complication of a dizzy spell or confusion, the need for vitamin A is increased. Some of the sources of vitamin A include cod liver oil, cereals and milk that is fortified, orange and yellow vegetables and fruits, and foods that contain beta-carotene such as broccoli and spinach.

Vitamin B, although constituting 12 different subtypes, are vital vitamins based on its wide range of effects that it has throughout the body. Having a direct impact on the body's energy levels, cell metabolism and brain function, ensuring that you take in all of the different types of vitamin B will ensure promotion in your cell health, as well as the stimulation and growth of your red blood cells. How this becomes important within the long COVID-19 framework is based on the breathlessness that long COVID-19 can present with. By stimulating an increase in the production of red blood cells by eating foods that contain a variety of the different vitamin B types, you are increasing the oxygen-carrying capacity of your body, decreasing the severity of the breathlessness, as well as its impact on your daily functioning. Sources of the different vitamin B subtypes are generally found in milk, eggs, liver and kidney, chicken and red meats, dark green vegetables, as well as tuna and salmon.

Iron is also very important to include in one's diet, as a lack of it can mimic some of the symptoms associated with long COVID-19. With a lack of iron resulting in anemia and a decrease in the oxygen-carrying capacity of blood, you will be left feeling severely fatigued. It is recommended that in a post-viral illness, between 10 to 15 milligrams of iron should be ingested every day. A lack of iron can cause headaches, brittle nails, as well as mimic the pins and needles that are typically felt as a possible symptom of long COVID-19. Beans, lentils, dark green and leafy vegetables, tofu and baked potatoes, are foods that contain relatively high levels of iron.

When focussing on the good nutrients and foods that are needed to bring your body back to its normal functioning, it is important that we steer clear from specific foods. Just because you are eating the good stuff, it does not mean you can run wild with fast foods. It is important to completely cut out the presence of any refined sugars in your diet as they promote inflammation in the body, negatively impacting the ability of your white blood cells to function effectively.

Alcohol and caffeinated beverages are an absolute no-no, primarily because they promote dehydration, which is ultimately what you are trying to avoid. Although you may have heard that orange juices and tomato soup are the best things to have when sick, they will actually do more harm than good. Their acidic nature aggravates the dysequilibrium present in your gut, resulting in an increase in pain and irritability. Avoiding salty foods is an absolute must when one is dealing with a post-viral illness. The reason for this is that the salt, in collaboration with any food items that contain fructose corn syrup and soybean oil, contributes to the inflammatory processes which make a large dent in your rate of recovery.

Supplements can play a pivotal role in diminishing and even ameliorating the symptoms that are associated with long COVID-19. Supplements become important when we are looking at the patient as a holistic entity. For example, a person with long COVID-19 may be a vegetarian due to their religion, which means that if other food sources for a specific vitamin or mineral cannot be sourced, taking a supplement is the next best option. Ensuring that one takes a good multivitamin is vital, as the chances of taking in all the amounts and types of minerals and vitamins each day, is rare and unrealistic. Taking a vitamin B complex tablet can ensure that your vitamin B levels remain normal, in order to aid with your body's restorative processes. Vitamin C supplements, coupled with that of an iron supplement is important especially for those that do not eat red meats. With vitamin C increasing the absorption of iron that is ingested, the result is both an increase in vitamin C and iron.

What it is important to take note of is where you plan on obtaining your protein from if you are tending towards using a supplement. The first place that many looking for a protein supplement will look is that of the protein powders, similar to those that gym-goers use. However, many erroneously use these protein shakes as a complete meal replacement. This is where the error comes in. Protein shakes can be convenient, however all the extra additives. If you are not educated about the different types of protein powders available, you may be at risk of harming your kidneys even while you are fighting long COVID-19. The presence of dextrins, artificial sweeteners, casein and whey protein concentrate provide negative nutrient effects, primarily because they block the absorption of some essential minerals and vitamins. This is why it is important that one rather substitutes the protein powder with higher protein content foods in your meal. For example, eating Greek yogurt in the morning with muesli and fruit provides so much more protein than a normal breakfast of cereal and milk.

It is important that when one who is progressing through long COVID-19 is not sure of what food to eat or what supplements to take (as well as avoid), that a healthcare professional is consulted. As soon as you become comfortable with asking about information that troubles you or that you are concerned about, you will be able to take ownership of what you are putting into your body. Nutrients and supplements are important however, only if they're of a high quality and they're used correctly.

CHAPTER 10

ANXIETY MANAGEMENT

"A crust eaten in peace is better than a banquet partaken in anxiety."
—Aesop fable

There is a specific level of fear that is associated with possibly contracting the coronavirus. What escalates this fear is that when you believe you have fought it successfully, you are made aware of the possibility that you could have long COVID-19. This feeling of fear is potentiated even further by the symptoms of mind fog and the decrease of mental alertness that are associated with long COVID-19. Extra precautions then need to be taken, especially if you are one who is living with an anxiety disorder. It is okay to feel frightened in light of the pandemic, especially as there is a high level of uncertainty circulating with questions that include, "When is this going to end?"

It is important to stay informed, especially to see what is happening in your community. We believe that each city should have support groups available for people that have long COVID-19, so that their anxiety can be shared amongst others going through the same situation. However, one needs to be careful about the number of times the news is checked, especially if you have just started your long COVID-19 recovery journey. Safety precautions, especially those that are bound to be excessive, as well as the constant levels of misinformation making its rounds, will only unnecessarily cause a spike in your anxiety levels. In terms of managing your fear and anxiety, there are a few measures that you can take in order to minimize the impact that the media has on your mental wellbeing. These are as follows:

• It is important that you stick to trustworthy sources that provide constant updates that are unbiased. Some examples of sources that you could focus on include that of the Center for Disease Control (CDC), the World Health Organization (WHO), as well as your local healthcare authorities. Many of these sources are starting to acknowledge long COVID-19 as a complication, leading to treatment modalities for the symptoms being made widely available.

• You should limit the number of times that you check the media for updates, as well as the online sources for content regarding long COVID-19. When one is quick to monitor the social media feeds, the action turns into a compulsive one which yields a counterproductive result. When you are unable to find any updates regarding long COVID-19, your mind will start to catastrophize situations, fueling your anxiety instead of alleviating it.

• Switch your phone off and give yourself a break from social media, especially if you start to feel overwhelmed. Having long COVID-19 can be especially taxing on one's mental health, primarily because it is not mentioned as much as the conventional COVID-19 virus. However, if your anxiety levels spike uncontrollably, allow yourself time periods to look for any updates.

• Some may find it a lot better to avoid social media and the internet entirely. What you can do is find someone that you trust and ask them to share updates with you once they become available.

Sometimes when you are unable to rationalize aspects that are out of your control, it is best to shift your mindset towards what you can control. As an individual that has long COVID-19, you can control how you feel about the illness, the preventative measures that you institute, as well as the extent you want to go to curb the symptoms you are experiencing. You also have control over how much you allow your anxiety to influence your daily life during long COVID-19.

We then ask the question, "How will we know whether we are feeling anxious?" This question is difficult to give a direct answer, primarily because those that have underlying anxiety will say that the symptoms differ from person to person. However, there are definitely some physical and mental symptoms that are directly associated with having anxiety. With regards to the physical symptoms, one with anxiety may present with a faster heartbeat, one that is more noticeable and that you can feel in your ears, you may even feel lightheaded and dizzy, coupled with headaches, a loss in your appetite and on the more severe scale, chest pains. Mental symptoms that are typical of anxiety include a feeling of being tense or nervous, worrying about the present, past or future, not being able to sleep, as well as a general feeling of being unable to relax.

However, these mental and physical changes play a pivotal role in altering the behaviors of those that have anxiety. How one would typically react in this situation is by not being able to enjoy their leisure time, having problems when needing to concentrate on a task, as well as having difficulty looking after themselves. This presentation is what can alert other individuals to elevated anxiety levels in others. What we like to say is that there are specific dos and don'ts that are associated with anxiety, especially in the time of long COVID-19.

Some of the dos include being able to talk to your friends and family about how you feel. Health professionals or counselors are more than willing to discuss your feelings with you, as well as provide you with solutions in order to overcome any negative effects that your feelings are having on you. There are even hotlines like that of the Samaritans which provide a free calling service for anyone that just wants to talk about their emotions with somebody else. Breathing exercises can also be used in order to center yourself and calm your emotions, with a positive being that they enable you to obtain a better quality of sleep. Exercise can be seen as a very positive means in relieving anxiety however do not forget to go nice and slow at the beginning, with a focus on not overexerting yourself. There are quite a few free mental wellbeing audio guides available online, which coupled with relaxation and mindfulness apps by the NHS apps library, will really aid in making you feel calmer in anxious situations.

Feeling anxious is not just caused by a single entity, especially when you have long COVID-19. It is because the symptoms affect different facets of your life that any anxiety you feel will potentiate. Having long COVID-19 impacts your ability to work, with a knock-on effect on your financial position. Having long COVID-19 may even hinder the relationships that you have with family and friends as some may find it difficult to understand what long COVID-19 is. This is why we say that the anxiety that is associated with long COVID-19 may not be directly due to the illness itself, but the knock-on effects that the illness has on other domains in your life.

For now, let us take you out of the picture for a second. The reason we do this is that we want you to equip you with the tools to also help someone else that may be suffering from anxiety due to long COVID-19. The first step is knowing how to identify the symptoms of someone with anxiety which, adding on from above, may also include nausea, being short of breath (exacerbated by long COVID-19), and profuse sweating. These feelings are characteristically accompanied by thought processes where one will believe the worst will happen. They will also tend to worry persistently, as well as have an all-or-none thinking pattern. It is when people start to overgeneralize (i.e., make broad assumptions based on a single event) that one should be cognizant of an impending bout of anxiety.

A clear demarcation needs to be made between what an anxious thought is, as well as how to identify an anxious behavior. The previous paragraph focused on anxious thoughts however, anxious behaviors are easier to identify because of their physical nature. Someone who is displaying features of anxiety may avoid situations they fear, second-guess all of their thought processes, become very irritable and frustrated when confronted with situations that they fear, and even tend to seek reassurance on their decisions. These thought processes are common in someone that has long COVID-19 as you are thrust into a post-viral illness that you may never have even known existed.

It is important to provide validation to those that suffer from anxiety. One of the worst possible sentences you could say to someone who has anxiety is, "Why are you getting upset over something that doesn't even directly affect you?" We need to make sure that we do not belittle the emotions that a person with anxiety is feeling. Instead, what you could do is ask how you are able to support them through moments where they are feeling anxious. You further want to ensure that you express genuine concern. Sometimes, all a person with anxiety wants to hear is that there is someone that wants to talk to them, that genuinely wants to know what is wrong. This can mean the world to someone that suffers from anxiety, and may even prompt them to open up about how long COVID-19 is making them feel, the fears as well as the uncertainty. This established dialogue may even result in the anxious person acknowledging that they need help or support in order to effectively cope during this time of recovery.

It is important to note that enabling anxiety as well as forcing confrontation will note end well for an anxious person. We need to acknowledge one's feelings, accepting them as being valid, and ensuring that they have support structures that they can rely on. Whether you are the one progressing through your long COVID-19 journey, or you know of someone else that is, make them feel loved and valued.

Anxiety is real, and the worst we can do is brush it under the carpet and pretend as if it doesn't exist.

CHAPTER 11

MINDFULNESS AND WELLBEING

"It is a curious thought, but it is only when you see people looking ridiculous that you realize just how much you love them."
–Agatha Christie

Having long COVID-19, or any other post-viral illness, is bound to make someone's stress, anxiety and depression rise to levels they may not have thought to be previously possible. However, learning how to cope with stress and depression in a healthy way, allows you as an individual to grow stronger as an individual, rising up to the challenge of not letting long COVID-19 dictate your life's direction. Stress and depression are expected emotions, especially in light of the pandemic. Social distancing can make you feel isolated and lonely, adding fuel to the fire regarding the severity of your stress and depression.

How stress and depression manifest during long COVID-19 is very typical of how any disease outbreak has the potential to make you feel. Examples of what you may feel include the following:

• An increased fear and worry about your own health. With long COVID-19, one stresses about whether you are going to recover from long COVID-19 unscathed, or whether the reason that you are going through long COVID-19 is due to an underlying medical condition. These are all real concerns to have about long COVID-19. These worries extend even further towards the health of your loved ones. If you didn't show symptoms during your initial COVID-19 infection, you wonder whether you may have unconsciously passed on the virus.

• You start to develop a change in sleeping and eating patterns. This happens because your mind is running wild with your current financial situation, questions that surround whether you will have a job once you have fully recovered, and even how you are going to make sure the work around the house gets done whilst you are still recovering.

• One may show an increase in the use of tobacco or alcohol as they are used to these substances helping them deal with stressful situations. This becomes problematic, especially regarding the impact that long COVID-19 already has on the organs of the body (more specifically the lungs).

Everyone will react to stressful situations differently. This is why there is no one-size-fits-all approach when dealing with stress and depression. This means that we need to provide solutions that prevent stress in a manner that allows adaptation to fit each individual's unique scenario. Stress has the ability to take its toll on anyone, especially those that may feel helpless during their long COVID-19 recovery.

We definitely recommend preventing stress through practicing positive self-talk coupled with taking mental breaks. As soon as we are able to replace our negative thoughts with that of positive thoughts, we will start to notice a shift in our mental health. A manner in which many individuals perform this task is by putting their stress into perspective. They ask themselves whether their current situation warrants as much stress as you are giving it. By trying to have a positive outlook on your current situation you are allowing yourself to cope through difficult times more effectively. With that being said, it is also important to allow your mind time to rest and recover. When we do not rest, our brain will not recover from the stress, leading to a build-up and ultimately exacerbated effects. Taking time to avoid situations that induce stress, whether it be online meetings or other people, is pivotal to being mentally and emotionally strong enough to facilitate a quicker recovery to long COVID-19.

Exercise seems to be good for anxiety, as well as for instances that cause stress. Although one mind it difficult to be exercising during long COVID-19, it is biologically and scientifically proven that 30 minutes of exercise (or as much as you can do) improves one's mood (thanks to the dopamine surge), as well as assists in creating a positive outlook on your physical and mental health. Moreover, performing exercise makes you feel less fatigued in the long run, increasing your concentration and establishing an improved sense of cognitive capabilities. As soon as you are able to see yourself in a positive light, you will begin to see that external and internal factors will not have as great an effect on you regarding the amount of stress you experience.

We tend to not give as much credit to the effects of putting one's thoughts down on paper. When you write down your thoughts, feelings and emotions, you are being real with yourself, helping you deal with your stress. Many individuals have a journal that they use to express their emotions, what they are struggling with and how their journey through long COVID-19 is making them feel. What this enables you to do is quantify your feelings of stress to the experiences that you have had, making you realize (in most cases) that you were stressing too much for a given scenario. This allows you to fill the time you would've used for stress, with that of activities that promote a positive wellbeing.

On the flip side, dealing with depression whilst going through long COVID-19 can prove to be of immense difficulty. You already feel like you don't want to do anything, now with the added effects of long COVID-19 it is not uncommon for one to fall even deeper into the pit of depression. However, dealing with depression during long COVID-19 is possible, and there are manners that can help you get out of the depression mindset.

We cannot emphasize the need of staying connected enough. Especially in times where you feel isolated, use technology to interact with your loved ones. You may not have the energy to go to your local coffee shop, but that doesn't mean that you can't invite someone over for a coffee. You will be able to gauge your energy levels based on which point you are at with your long COVID-19 recovery. Dropping people a text message, setting up a video call, or even playing a video game online together not only makes one feel connected, but brings a sense of joy that isn't common during a pandemic.

We have heard the saying "you are not alone" and we have yet to hear words that are more true. The harsh reality is that people believe that they are alone, in their health problems, in their finances, in their relationships with their parents. However, this is where it is important to join a support group, both for depression and for long COVID-19. Being amongst others that have depression, even if it is virtual, makes you feel that you aren't as isolated as you once thought. This is where you will also be encouraged to both give and receive advice on how to cope with having a post-viral illness and still dealing with the depression of facing each day with a positive outlook.

Depression can be alleviated by reminding yourself that there are times of joy in life. Whether that means getting a pet that you can look after, taking your neighbor's pet for a walk, or spending a few hours reading your favorite childhood book, different folks will have different tasks that boost their mood. You need to make time to enjoy the fun activities, to allow yourself to explore possible new hobbies, or expand on old ones. The realism behind your long COVID-19 recovery journey is that it may be long, so you might as well try to enjoy it.

Cognitive brain therapy (CBT) is used as a mainstay of treatment for depression, focusing on your negative thoughts regarding long COVID-19 and replacing them with healthier ones. As CBT starts to make you aware of these thoughts, you are able to positively alter them to represent your mind's true intentions. When regressing into a spiral of depression, the thoughts that are altered using CBT halt the progression of your spiral, altering your attitude towards your depression whilst allowing you to feel capable of taking control of your mental health.

Many individuals have used a wellness toolbox in order to reclaim a sense of positivity in their lives, especially in light of long COVID-19. When you reclaim your positivity, you are reminding yourself what it feels like to feel joy, happiness and self-love, reminding yourself that these emotions do exist in the world, despite what you are going through. These toolboxes may differ from person to person, based on what they enjoy, however, starting off by listing ten such mood boosters and performing them regularly will aid in that paradigm shift into a more positive outlook on your long COVID-19 journey. An example of a wellness toolbox can include the following:

• Pick up your favorite book, make a nice cup of herbal tea and spend some time in nature.

• List some things that you like about yourself.

• Ask some friends and family for funny TV shows or movies (or whichever genre you enjoy).

• Listen to the newest album of your favorite artist or band.

• Schedule an online conference call with your closest group of friends.

• Enjoy a nice hot bath with candles in order to make you feel relaxed.

- Start scrapbooking the best experiences in your life thus far.

- Spend some quality time with your pet.

- Ask your friends or family to choose a puzzle that best describes you, and then invite them to build it with you.

We cannot deny that there are going to be bouts of depression, anxiety and stress when journeying through long COVID-19. However, we can choose to look at the negative aspects, or we can learn to shift our mindsets to focus on the positives. There are so many activities that you can incorporate into your life as your recovery continues. There was nothing that said that the recovery has to be boring, and the possible activities that we mentioned above are proof of that.

3

Learning to Live With Long COVID-19

Contents:

CHAPTER 12

RUNNING YOUR HOME

"There is a homely adage which runs: 'Speak softly and carry a big stick; you will go far.'"
—Theodore Roosevelt

With the effects that long COVID-19 has on your health, energy levels, and mental health, running your home can seem like a daunting task. We acknowledge, especially those of you that have kids, that running a house before you had long COVID-19 was hard enough. However, how do we explain to our loved ones that we just don't have the energy that is necessary to move around like we used to? This is where it is important to have open communication with your family and friends. However hard it may be, it is a necessary conversation to have.

It is in this manner that we want to provide you with some tips for healthy and open communication with your loved ones regarding your experiences and emotions with long COVID-19. Our tips are as follows:

• Finding the right time is important. You want to make sure that your loved ones are fully attentive to the emotions that you are conveying to them. It is finding time when everyone is calm and not distracted by work or household tasks, to talk about your worries, concerns and feelings.

• Some individuals that are going through long COVID-19 may find it difficult to have a face to face conversation with their loved ones. If it is not possible, then scheduling a video call to speak to everyone may be a better option. If you feel like having a crowd of individuals would be too much, focus on individually setting up a time with the respective people. You want to make sure that what you are saying is understood and not misinterpreted. This is done in order to prevent any possibility of there being a miscommunication.

• Being honest with your loved ones about your recovery with long COVID-19 is of utmost importance. If this means that you end up crying, then that is okay. You need to ensure that the seriousness of your emotions is explained succinctly so that everyone can understand what you are going through.

It is well known that your needs may change as your symptoms change during long COVID-19. This is why it is important to have check-in sessions with your loved ones, to let them know how you are doing, including both the physical and mental aspects. It is also important that you voice your concerns as soon as they arise instead of bottling them all up and informing your loved ones about everything all at once.

Thinking about the life that your partner and family need to live should be taken into consideration. Maybe now that you cannot work your partner or housemates need to take up extra shifts to cover the rent. We need to encourage a two-way conversation that is expressed honestly. We also need to be cognizant of the lives of others. This means that we cannot expect one person to now operate in the capacity of two, there needs to be a form of understanding between the two parties. Although, it is understandable that during your recovery with long COVID-19, that you won't be able to do as many tasks as usual, expressing your thanks to your loved one for their aid really goes a long way in making them feel appreciated.

A very important, yet difficult decision that needs to be made is based on the foods that you are to consume throughout your recovery period. These foods may differ entirely from what you and your family are used to eating and can even put some strain on your loved ones as they don't know exactly what it is you need. What we recommend is the setting up of a food calendar, where you not only write down all the ingredients for each dish, but also any alternatives that can be purchased. This will not only remove any stress that is felt by your loved ones when doing grocery shopping, but it also allows you to incorporate variety into your eating. What many have found helpful is sharing their list with a dietitian for approval–just to ensure that their choices are adequately nutritious for optimal recovery.

Seeking aid from your loved ones is especially important when you need to focus on the quality of sleep that you are getting. Poor sleep, even in the light of a post-viral illness, will both unnecessarily prolong your recovery time but will also increase the intensity of your anxiety, stress and depression. This is why sleep management plans need to be clearly communicated to your loved ones. These strategies include the possible use of medications (upon prescription by your healthcare professional) to aid in obtaining sound and good quality sleep. A very important factor would also be one's sleep environment. It is important that one's environment be as quiet as possible in order to obtain uninterrupted sleep. This means that your loved ones need to ensure that you are allowed to obtain this sleep as it will only be to your benefit in your recovery process.

Now as an individual that is taking care of someone that has long COVID-19, what is there that you can do? With the needs already being clarified, it may be worthwhile to take on some of the small practical tasks in order to ensure that their energy levels are not diminished. Some of the examples of what you can do to help them, are the following:

• Make a healthy meal for the one that has long COVID-19. Even if you aren't the best chef, the fact that you tried will definitely put a smile on their face, as well as will contribute towards them having a positive mental state.

• One of the worst images to wake up to is that of dirty dishes in the sink. So, why not ensure that your sick household member does not need to even look at the sight by washing up the dishes every evening.

• Ensuring that there is always transport to their medical appointments is a manner of not only showing you care, but also showing that you want to be actively involved in the recovery process.

• Helping look after the kids, or offering to feed the pets is another task that will leave the ill household member feeling grateful and more relaxed.

• Doing the grocery shopping, returning library books and picking up any other essentials are all outside tasks that need to be done by a loved one. The one who is ill cannot stay awake in her own house, getting her outside to run errands will not end well for either party.

• Do not fear asking your children to help out with the chores or with running errands. If your children are old enough, this may even be the perfect opportunity for them to learn some life skills. It really is a win-win situation.

There are many tasks that one can do in order to make sure long COVID-19 does not infiltrate any friend, family or romantic dynamics as it has the potential to do so. As long as there is an agreement with regards to what another can do to help, the recovery process for long COVID-19 should be a lot smoother.

A typical worry that one has is the financial burden that long COVID-19 will place on their lives as well as on their household. This can be very stressful, especially if your workplace and employers are not as understanding of your situation as you would've liked them to be. Many countries have what they call "statutory sick pay" which an ill individual may qualify for. In the United Kingdom this form of payment will pay up to 28 weeks if you were previously employed but are now unable to work.

As you are progressing through your recovery it is important that the attempt is still made to have some quality time with your loved ones. It is in this way that you can let them know how appreciative you are of their help. At this point, when you start to regain your energy levels, you can begin increasing the quality time that you provide for your loved ones. For some this may mean eating one of the three meals at the table as a family, for others it may be getting out of bed and watching a movie with a loved one.

Whenever and wherever you can, it is important to do things that you enjoy. When we spoke about having mindfulness breaks and filling these breaks with joy, we really meant it. One who is ill does not want to have an atmosphere that is dull, dreary and places on into a deeper form of depression. Whilst one is ill, it doesn't mean that you need to stop cultivating your own happiness. The impact that it has on a family environment when the ill person is trying their best to be happy despite their illness, makes everyone feel that they are able to overcome this tough and trying time together.

CHAPTER 13

RETURNING TO WORK

"Life is for living and working at. If you find anything or anybody a bore, the fault is in yourself."

—Queen Elizabeth I of England

J ust the thought of needing to return to work after having battled through long COVID-19 can evoke intense anxiety and stress. These feelings are completely valid as we have no idea whether we will be capable to fulfill the needs of our job once we return, or how long it will take to reach one's normal state of efficacy. This is why one needs to be sure that one is physically, mentally and emotionally ready to return to the workplace, or either to resume work from home.

If you feel that the physical demands of returning to work are out of your reach, try reaching out to your employer regarding the phased return to work by working from home. The benefit of working from home is that it will help avoid exposure to other colds and viruses which would compound post-viral fatigue. Having progressed through long COVID-19, there is a high chance that your immune system is not as strong as you are used to it being. Thus, by being able to save time and conserve energy by not commuting to work, you are able to spend this time on strengthening your immune system by exercising and cooking nutritious meals.

Research is still grey with regards to a direct time period when those with long COVID-19 should be eligible to return to work. However, some governments have released pamphlets saying that if one is clear of symptoms for 14 days then they can phase in their return to work. Other leaflets state that if you have long COVID-19 and an underlying condition which includes cancer or having had an organ transplant in the past, you will need to self-isolate for 12 weeks before the phased return to work.

Once you have decided that you will return, there are probably a few things you should prepare for. Other than needing to have discussions with your employers regarding your work roles and working hours, here are a few extra considerations that you should think of:

> • Ready yourself for some paperwork. During the period right before you begin work again, take some time to take a read through the company's sick leave policies. This is done in order to ensure that you are aware of any supporting documentation that may be required. Most of the time one would require medical clearance from a qualified doctor stating that your health will not be compromised should you choose to return to work.

> • Some employers are not as understanding as others, this is why it is a good idea to do a brief read through your rights as

an employee. For example, in the UK you are entitled to compensation whether your leave from work is due to stress, mental health issues or complications from other illnesses. Another example is in the United States where some companies are subject to the Family and Medical Leave Act which allows up to 12 weeks of unpaid leave for specific medical conditions.

• Readying yourself for the day of work will require you to ensure you get a good night of sleep the night before your return. Having gotten used to the 12-hour sleeping pattern that was needed for your body to recover from long COVID-19, the worry of being ready for work on time can induce unnecessary levels of anxiety. If you need to leave the house and return to an office, you will most likely have forgotten about the travel time needed, so it is important to make sure you leave early enough.

• Go easy on yourself! The effects of long COVID-19 may still be lingering slightly since you have decided to return to work. This is why it is important to not put a large amount of undue pressure on yourself as you phase yourself back into the working world. Do not expect yourself to work at 110% when you feel closer to 40%. Allow yourself that extra time to read through your requirements, to answer those emails, taking breaks when you feel it is necessary. The worst thing you can do is cause yourself to burn out on the first day back. You may have a backlog of emails, meetings and apologies that you have to send. Take all these tasks one step at a time and in a time that you feel comfortable with.

- Remember, you have the support from human resources upon your return. When you were off from work you felt isolated and vulnerable. Fast track to your first day back you may feel overwhelmed by the number of people in your virtual meetings, or by the number of people at the office. It is important to look after your mental health during this time. Whether it be obtaining emotional support from a friend, or needing to talk about readjusting your workload, getting in contact with your human resources department may be a good first step.

Once you have phased in your return to work, you may feel that the workload you have been given is a lot in comparison to before you had COVID-19. However, you need to remember that you have not been in the rhythm of working for quite some time, which would impact your ability to work effectively. However, this is where we can implement the 3 Ps very effectively. Pacing yourself becomes key when you return to work, especially when implementing breaks when you feel tired. If you are working from home, make an active effort to give yourself a 15-minute break for every one hour that you work, whether it be drinking a cup of herbal tea or taking a quick walk in the garden.

Planning your work schedule for the day is important, primarily because you will need to make sure that you have achieved all your outcomes by the end of the day. This is where prioritizing becomes important as you cannot work from the furthest date to the most current, as then you will miss out on the latest work that needs to be completed. For example, if you were off sick for six weeks, it would be more to your benefit to answer meeting requests from two days ago than those from five weeks ago.

Getting your employer to understand your reasoning for requiring a phased return into the workplace may prove to be a bit more difficult than one would think. If once explaining how you felt, the emotions that accompanied long COVID-19, as well as the worries regarding financial stability and the ability to return to work, your employer still does not understand, try getting your treating healthcare professional to rationally explain long COVID-19 to your employer. Sometimes when we allow our treating healthcare professionals to explain the medical situations, it provides some form of weighted context to your illness claim. However, it is in this way that we suggest scheduling a meeting with your employer, one where there are no external distractions so that you have their full attention when explaining long COVID-19 to them.

You won't be able to convince all your work colleagues to be empathetic once you return. Unfortunately, that is just how people are. However, what you can do is let the coworkers that you feel closest to, as well as your supervisor, know about your phased return and that you may need help in being able to return to your full capacity. By writing your needs down and communicating this to them either via face to face contact, or via email, is a fantastic start to the conversation, especially because you are making them aware that you may need some help from time to time.

During this time of COVID-19, especially for those that have progressed into long COVID-19, the stress associated with the possibility of receiving a pay cut or being retrenched can weigh heavily on one's mental health. However, this is not an uncommon feeling and should not be brushed aside as it is a real and valid concern to have. But the question arises, "How does one survive financial stress?" Getting through a rough financial patch is a normal occurrence and a part of life. However there definitely are manners to help you in surviving this period of financial stress. Some of these methods include the following:

• Ensure that you are staying active. By this we mean that you shouldn't let having financial stresses impact your ability to feel happy. Continue making visits to see your friends, do that free online course to boost your CV, and try your best to continue paying the bills. If you find that you have more time at home either because you are working from home or are working fewer hours, try to implement a fun gym routine. There are so many free fitness plans online that will definitely contribute to you saving some money as you won't need to pay any gym subscriptions.

• Learn to face your fears when you are starting to deal with potential debt. It is never too late to start obtaining advice regarding how to prioritize and organize your finances efficiently and effectively. It is human nature for individuals to avoid conversation when they feel overly anxious. If you know that you are spending too much money on takeout whilst you are fighting long COVID-19 then focus on substituting those takeout meals with fresh, nutritional and cheaper alternatives from your local supermarket.

• Focus on avoiding alcohol. Even though it is advised that

you do not consume alcohol when recovering from long COVID-19 (as it potentiates dehydration), as well as when you are having financial difficulties. Some people may use alcohol as a manner to numb the pain associated with the emotions of financial insecurity, as well as helping make time pass quicker. However, alcohol on the flip side will potentiate your stress levels whilst not helping your wallet, a rather counterproductive approach to handling your money.

• Make sure that you do not sacrifice your daily routine. What we mean by this is that you should live as normally as you possibly can. The downside if this is not achieved is that your mental health will take a dip, leading to the potentiation of symptoms associated with depression.

• Do not be afraid to ask for help. There are legal governmental organizations that help you to regulate your cash flow and start paying your debts without compromising on your livelihood. For example, the NHS has the Money Advice Service and national Debtline that provide aid in finance regulation.

As you can see from this chapter, it can be a very daunting task having to return to work. people are going to have questions about where you were and why it took you so long to return. You are most probably going to be explaining the same story until you are blue in the face, however it is all a part of the process. Remember, your mental health comes first. Do not feel embarrassed that you need to work at a slower pace than what you are used to. Take it as your body telling you that it can work, but that it just needs a bit more time.

CHAPTER 14

REACHING OUT TO OTHERS

"Selfishness is not living as one wishes to live, it is asking others to live as one wishes to live."

—Oscar Wilde

A sense of pride is typically what stops us from reaching out to others. We fear that we are imposing ourselves on their lives when that may not be the case. We fear that we are making our problems theirs, and because we don't know what they are going through, we don't know how our worries would affect them. These are a few thought processes that cross one's mind when they either think about or are told to reach out to others for help.

Long COVID-19 is an illness that ebbs and flows, meaning that some days we are going to feel better or worse than others. This means that when you are at your worst you may feel that there is nobody that understands you or even wants to hear about your issues. When you start to feel this severe sense of isolation, it is one of the signs that you should possibly think about receiving professional treatment. There are so many other signs that lead to you needing to possibly attend therapy. Primarily, most of these instances are based on alterations in your mood, levels of productivity and your behavior. It is when these stressful moments and changes persist for longer than two weeks (which could be even longer in terms of the symptoms that present as a part of long COVID-19) that action should be taken. Here are a few of the other signs that you can spot for yourself:

• Hopelessness: This specific emotion becomes very important to identify because as soon as you feel there is no hope and that you are worthless within your community and at what you do, you are stepping into depression territory. Practical examples that can be seen as precipitations of hopelessness include that of worrying that you do not have a future, that there is no way that you are going to be successful, and that you do not deserve to be happy. These feelings coupled with not feeling motivated to positively influence your current situation, are definite signs that therapy should be sought out.

• Constant worrying: It is absolutely normal for humans to worry in small doses however, when the worrying becomes excessive, the worry then becomes a barrier that stops you from enjoying your life. With this constant sense of worry developing into anxiety, physical symptoms which include headaches and stomach aches can precipitate.

• Appetite and sleeping pattern disturbances: As soon as you start to notice that you are constantly tired, more so than with that which is experienced with long COVID-19 you can rest assured that your mental health is being negatively impacted.

Once deciding to attend therapy, in order to regulate your eating and sleeping patterns, cognitive behavioral therapy may be performed.

• Irritability: When recovering through long COVID-19, one needs to be consciously aware of one's levels of irritability. This irritability may precipitate into physical impatience when tasks take longer than they should.

• Loss of productivity: If you are struggling to work or focus at home, especially when you have multiple worry streams, you will find that your productivity starts to plummet. Once this happens you start to blame yourself, rendering yourself incompetent at being productive. Thus, you start to fall deeper into the pit of depression, emphasizing the need for immediate intervention.

• Worry from others: Sometimes we need to listen to the inputs that our loved ones speak to us about without automatically taking what they are saying as an attack. It can be easier for others to notice these changes in you as your mind is racing at 100 times its usual speed, thus it is normal for you not to notice. In this case what a loved one can do is to check-in regularly, approach the subject of therapy with due caution and sensitivity, to not assume what they are going through, as well as to constantly remind them that you have their unequivocal support.

Whilst it may be slightly easier to spot when you are spiraling into a depressive episode, how do we approach others regarding asking them for their assistance. Well, this can be tackled in one of two ways depending on your personality. You can either take the friendship route where you focus on asking for help from those that know you the best, that can relate to what you are doing, and that will be an open ear for you to talk to about your issues. Alternatively, you can take the professional route which encompasses booking an appointment with a therapist or joining an online support group. For some, they might find that incorporating both is more advantageous, whereby one would then attend the support groups but then have that extra support from your loved ones (whether this is your partner, friends or family) when the support group is not immediately accessible.

It is important to be open and honest with whoever you decide to talk to regarding your mental health. The reason for this is that you want them to understand the full reasoning behind your actions. You will only be able to benefit completely from their advice if you are going to be completely open and honest with them. This means that you should feel at liberty to express your worries, your concerns and even your fears. For those that you trust, you shouldn't feel the need to refrain from sharing anything.

THE SPIRAL OF NEGATIVITY

One of the common results from constantly being in environments and situations that are stressful and anxiety-inducing, is that you start to slip into a negative spiral of depression. It is in this spiral that you completely isolate yourself from everyone and everything, making your loved ones rather concerned about your physical and mental wellbeing. In order to distance oneself from this spiral of negativity, one can learn to gradually make mental shifts. What this means is that you are essentially stopping your negative thought processes in their tracks and substituting them with positive ones.

The manner in which this is done is by reflection on the current situation and choosing to focus on something else that is of greater importance. It is practically a gear shift that prevents the same negative situation from being stuck on a loop in your brain. However, what makes this difficult is that it may prompt you to unlearn some negative behaviors that you were unknowingly inherently taught. An example of this is developing a sense of stressful perfectionism from being in a top-performing school and needing to always be the best. We will now look at some of the modalities you can implement in order to prevent the possibility of a negative spiral occurring.

I SHOULD

The word 'should' is one that should be completely removed from one's vocabulary, especially if they suffer from depression or are currently fighting through long COVID-19. The reason for this is that using the word 'should' triggers a sense of guilt that can cause a high level of frustration to occur, resulting in the initiation of the negativity spiral. When we look at these 'should' statements, they tend to contribute negatively towards our anxiety in that it is setting up demands on our lives that we, at that time due to illness or mental health issues, will not be able to successfully complete.

As an example, if one says that they should be going to the gym every day, even though they know they haven't been to the gym in months, the spiral of negativity begins. However, if we were to alter that statement to say, "I will try my best to attend the gym every day. The way that I am going to do that is as follows…" then we are allowing ourselves the opportunity to put measures in place that allow us to achieve these demands without our mental health taking a dip.

WHAT IS CAUSING YOUR ANXIETY?

Only after repeatedly being in a toxic environment do we begin to realize that it is a source of anxiety, stress and depression. If you are aware that a specific situation is causing you to spiral, you should critically analyze the situation so that you can avoid all the elements that may even be present in other situations. You start off by asking who you were with, being open and honest with yourself regarding whether it was the person, their attitudes or actions that caused a spike in your anxiety levels. Establishing when and where the anxiety-inducing event took place provides context that could solidify an anxiety-inducing element. By completely removing yourself from all the identified elements, as well as that exact situation, you will completely ameliorate the chances of entering into a spiral of negativity.

WHAT MOOD DO YOU HAVE IN THIS SITUATION?

When you are able to understand how you are feeling from an emotional point of view, you are able to deal with your emotions head-on. If a situation makes you feel irritated, nervous, angry, and guilty, record these in a journal and rate the intensity of each one. What the main point of this activity is, is analyzing how much your thoughts are directly influenced by a specific range of moods.

WHAT ARE YOUR GO-TO THOUGHTS?

This specific aspect is the most important as you will begin to realize how much negative self-talk is involved when you are in a situation that spurs on negative moods. Some of the common thought processes that will run through your mind include thinking of the following statements:

- "I shouldn't even try because I am probably going to mess this up."

- "I don't even know why I try. I'm so dumb!"

- "I'm never going to find love. I'm going to end up alone."

- "The world is such an awful place because nobody likes me."

- "I cannot muster the strength to cope with these situations."

These statements can be seen as rather destructive thought processes, this is why we need to break tasks down so that we can effectively shift our mindset. We want to ensure that we shift our mindset away from the mood that is having the greatest impact on your thought processes. An example of this is tackling the statement, "There is no way I can do this, I am going to mess this up!" Evaluating this situation we need to place it into context. By breaking down your emotions and moods into direct causative scenarios, you are able to gain control of your emotions and prevent your emotions from taking control of your life.

CHALLENGE YOURSELF

It is important to understand that making a mental shift isn't about flipping onto the opposite extreme of a spectrum. One does not just make a simple decision in a sad situation and two seconds later you are happy. Coming to terms with the fact that sometimes, no matter how hard you will try to alter your thought patterns, there will be times that you will be unsuccessful in doing so. It is in these times that you should be satisfied with the progress that you have made. By having successfully acknowledged the destructive thought processes, you are already well on your way to being able to make that mental shift.

What makes challenging yourself so important is that it also allows you to realize that it is okay to sometimes feel sad. Being able to successfully establish a mental shift doesn't mean that you will no longer ever feel sadness. What it does mean is that you are able to recognize that there may be an unrealistic element at play which is causing your sadness, prompting you to work around the emotion and ameliorate its impact. Forcing positive thoughts is not helpful, even more so if you live with an underlying mental condition such as anxiety or depression. Also remember that it is okay to ask for professional help, especially when you are struggling to think in a positive manner.

One may also find that changing your focus can go a long way in ensuring that you do not fall into a negative spiral. When you are depressed, you begin to realize that all your thoughts and feelings first pass through a lens of negativity. Some people find that distracting themself in the midst of their spiral of negativity, tends to work. This means that you need to find a task that adds more purpose to your life than your depression, that brings you joy. We know that this may be immensely difficult, especially seeing as you are progressing through long COVID-19. It is in this way that you should be able to find some sources of joy and happiness that you can tap into when necessary. You cannot force yourself to have fun however, you can change and alter your immediate circumstances in order to make them a little less depressing. Whether you find that a walk in the garden, or listening to some uplifting music does the trick, the benefit that this will have on your mental health will be noticeable.

We find that allowing ourselves to not get into a negative spiral of thoughts will require a lot more work than we thought. However, we need to come to terms with when our health is not getting better, and be honest with ourselves about it. What many in the long COVID-19 support groups have done is that they give themselves a set time period, where if they still do not feel better they return to their healthcare professional. They do this separately for their physical and mental symptoms. For example, what someone may do is that when they feel 72 hours of constant depression, they contact their therapist the next morning to make an appointment.

It is not easy asking for help from others, especially when you are so used to being independent. However, what one needs to realize is that humans are caring creatures by nature, and will want to help their loved ones where they can. As you progress through long COVID-19, and even other areas of your life, you do not need to let depression, anxiety and your mental health get the better of you. You have the potential and information to fight against your negative emotions, and what we can tell you is that the fight is definitely worth it.

CHAPTER 15

THE R.I.S.E PROTOCOL

"Reality is something you rise above."

–Anon

B ouncing back after going through an illness as taxing as long COVID-19 can prove to be difficult. However, our bodies are made of regenerative tissue and have all the capabilities that are necessary in order to bounce back after an illness. With that being said there are definitely a few methods that you can employ in order to ensure that you are getting back into your routine in a manner that is not mentally or physically taxing to yourself and those in your immediate surroundings.

It is important that you take your time when regaining momentum in your life. If you push yourself too hard and too fast you will crash a lot harder than when you were ill. Biologically this will result in an even weaker immune system that predisposes you to an array of other infections. If you were used to going for a run every morning before long COVID-19, then start off with a small walk. One needs to be mindful of how our bodies feel and pace ourselves accordingly.

Journaling on its own can be seen as a rather relaxing task however, it becomes even more important when you are bouncing back from an illness. When you write down how you are coping with your integration back towards a state of normality, you are able to grade and quantify your integration back into society. It is very difficult to not think of all the work that you have missed whilst you have been on your long COVID-19 recovery journey. However, you are only going to negatively impact yourself and your emotions by stressing about it, especially when all your cognitive efforts should be focused on getting better. Research shows that writing down what you should and want to do when you feel better gives you the motivation to make the correct and healthier choices, resulting in a decreased recovery time.

Your energy levels may result in you hardly responding to anyone, which is understandable. However, not everyone that emails you, texts you or gives you a call needs your undivided and immediate attention or response. Being open and honest with these individuals is important, especially if you occupy quite an important position in the workplace and people rely on your insight and decision-making skills. Remember, everyone has been sick at one or stages of their lives, they will most likely (and will need to) understand.

It is important to wind down during the evening. By this we mean that you should turn off all electronic screens a good 90 minutes before you are due to fall asleep. It is so easy for those who are ill with long COVID-19 to rely more on their phones as a means of remaining integrated with society that we forget about the large amounts of blue light that is emitted from these devices. Blue light causes strain on our eyes, with research also linking it to both physical and mental fatigue, which one really doesn't need anymore whilst progressing through recovery from long COVID-19. You may find it that much easier to binge-watch every TV series you have been recommended, and unnecessarily open Instagram every five minutes however, by turning off your devices you are allowing yourself the time for your own self-care as well as ensuring that your sleeping environment is adequate for a good night of rest.

The chances are that the amount of time that you have spent in bed during your recovery is a lot more than you probably have ever envisioned. We need to think about the constituents of our body at this point, with our muscles and joints starting to feel stiff as they haven't been used as much as they are used to. This is why it is important to stretch during your recovery period as a very sudden start can result in aches, pains and in some severe cases, injury. Starting with some long and slow stretches will allow your muscles to become accustomed to being back in operation.

R.I.S.E

We want to introduce a protocol that we have found to be pivotal in allowing you to get back into your best shape physically, mentally, emotionally and socially. The R.I.S.E protocol is very well known, and has been developed by Greta Steiner as a means for returning into a healthcare system. As we move through the different sections of the protocol, discussing them a bit more in-depth, we invite you to not think rigidly about what each subsection contains and to blend in your own unique modalities so as to customize the protocol to fit your personality.

ROUTINE

Having a routine that encompasses a perfect balance of rest and activity, is pivotal for those that are going through long COVID-19. Ensuring that you have this routine will further block the amounts of stress that you feel, as well as keep your sanity in check. Repetition is scientifically proven to be of benefit to your physical health, but can even improve your mental health by playing an active role in decreasing your stress levels.

Decisions are what allows us to add stress to our lives. We find that the more decisions we make, the more amounts of uncertainty we ingrain into our daily lives, leading to a lesser sense of self-control. Although decision-making forms a critical part of our lives, creating a regular rhythm, can remove most of the guesswork that you may need to resort to during your day.

Tel Aviv University has put in a lot of research in order to see the impact that having a predictable and repetitive routine has on the reduction of anxiety and keeping one calm. Routines will further ensure that you can take control of your day, and ultimately your life. The worst that we can do in the morning is to jump from task to task without any set structure, which is why a set routine should be made and you should stick with it. By maintaining a set schedule you are not allowing the probability of chance to seep into your life, which will ultimately result in a heightened concentration as well as less physical energy being consumed.

It is important to quantify the amount of energy that you have at the beginning of the day, and allocate these amounts of energy so that the most important tasks are completed first. For example, spending a great amount of energy on finishing important paperwork for your new job shows greater importance than making sure the grass outside has been wet sufficiently.

One of the main pitfalls regarding routines is that we do not enjoy personalizing our routines as we see it as too much work, rather opting to adopt somebody else's routine as it is seen as being less time-consuming. However, by adopting someone else's schedule you are not allowing enough time to finish specific tasks, especially when you are dealing with long COVID-19 over and above everything else that requires your time. What we would suggest is this: focus on removing as many variables as you possibly can.

We will use the example of getting ready for work in the morning and being indecisive regarding what you should wear. However, if you find that you have too many options, by removing any form of clutter, you are leading a lesser amount of decisions and thus decreasing the potential stress levels that can seep into your routines. When you focus on removing excess choices, you are effectively saving time and energy in the process. This further allows you to shift your focus towards other tasks that you may not have had the time or energy for before.

IMMUNITY

For those that are suffering from long COVID-19, they will find that there is a greater need for boosting the immune system in whatever way they can. However, the immune system is an immensely complicated smorgasbord of cells and molecules which can prove some difficulty in understanding how your body is reacting to the presence of illnesses. However, what we plan to do is lean towards a myth-buster approach to let you know some of the facts associated with your immune system.

A very common myth is that the more active that your immune system is, the healthier you are. We can already debunk this myth based on the effects of long COVID-19. As many have said, too much of a good thing can be detrimental. For example, when someone shows that they are allergic to something, our immune system jumps into overdrive. There is also a constant hyperactive immune response with some underlying conditions which include diabetes and arthritis.

Many individuals further believe that the more nutrients, irrespective of amounts, that you put into your body, the healthier your immune system will be. What is consistent with the evidence is that only a certain amount of vitamins can be stored within the body. The rest that is not absorbed is excreted in our urine. So, if you go over the recommended daily allowance of specific vitamins and minerals, there is no positive benefit thereof.

There are quite a few things that you can do in order to strengthen your immune system. Some examples of this include:

• Avoiding infection or extra illnesses by maintaining adequate hygiene practices. This includes washing your hands regularly and thoroughly, as well as ensuring that meat is adequately cooked.

• Ensure that you are up to date with your immunizations as they offer adequate protection against disease-causing organisms that our bodies may not be able to effectively fight on their own, especially in the context of having long COVID-19.

• Ensure that you do not smoke, do not drink alcohol and that your bodyweight is maintained. This will ensure that there are no extra complications of you having long COVID-19.

• With regards to your diet, one needs to make sure that the foods that you are taking in are high in fruits, whole grains and vegetables. One wants to ensure that the amount of saturated fat and sugar is restricted as much as possible. One needs to make sure that these restricted constituents do not take up more than 10% of your total calorie intake.

• A healthy body results in a healthy mind, this means that one, especially those with long COVID-19 should push to having approximately 150 minutes of exercise per week.

• What we highly recommend in terms of immunity, is that you go for a regular medical screening test in order to ensure that your body is still functioning well in light of long COVID-19.

The immunity of the human body is a complex yet efficient system. However, we want to ensure that we provide it with as much support as we possibly can in order to ensure our recovery rate is as short as possible. The stronger we make our immune system, the better we will be able to fight back against long COVID-19 as well as prevent any opportunistic infections from occurring.

SLEEP

Research has found that a good night of sleep is seen as being even more important than eating a healthy and balanced diet, and even exercising. This makes logical sense seeing as sleep regains our body's energy, and if we do not have any energy, the thought of making food and exercising will already drain your energy levels. Nowadays people are sleeping a lot less than they did in the past, coupled with the quality of sleep being very low. This not only leaves one grumpy in the morning, but it also ensures that you are not able to operate at your best in comparison to when you would've had a full eight hours of good quality sleep. If this has not convinced you, maybe the following benefits of sleep will:

> • In today's day and age many are bodyweight conscious. This could pose difficulty especially if your exercise levels are not what they should be during long COVID-19. Research has shown that there is a strong link between poor sleep and weight gain. There were extensive review studies conducted whereby it was found that children and adults with poor sleeping patterns were 89% and 55% more likely to develop obesity. It is said that it is based on hormone abnormalities and a decrease in motivation to exercise, due to tiredness, that potentiates the chances of developing obesity.

• We are still trying to figure out how this works, but it is said that sleep-deprived individuals are more likely to eat meals that have more calories. This is due to the fluctuations in appetite hormones (such as a reduction in the amount of leptin). One would hope that with long COVID-19 that sleep would not be a problem. However, one must remember that it is not the amount of sleep you get, but the quality of the sleep.

• Having good quality sleep has proven to maximize and im-prove concentration and problem-solving skills. A study that focused on medical interns showed that a lack of good quality sleep resulted in an increase in the number of medical errors by 36%.

• During long COVID-19 it is of utmost importance that we obtain good quality sleep in order to maximize the physical capabilities of our bodies during our illness. As one progresses through long COVID-19 a lack of sleep will result in a greater possibility and amount of functional impairments.

• A review of 15 studies has shown that individuals who do not get between seven and eight hours of good quality sleep, are at a greater risk of developing heart disease. In terms of long COVID-19 we would like to ensure that this does not become a possible complication.

• Individuals who are not getting at least six hours of good quality sleep per night are heightening their chances of devel-oping type 2 diabetes. Biologically this is due to the reduction in insulin sensitivity, causing the amount of sugar present in the bloodstream to increase.

• Having just spoken about our body's immunity, it is well known that sleep will improve our immune function. Research shows that individuals who sleep fewer than seven hours are up to three times more likely to fall prey to the common cold, than in comparison to those that got more than eight hours of sleep.

It is important that sleep is to be strengthened with the use of good nutrition, exercise and a positive mental health outlook. We cannot stress the importance of this, especially with someone that is progressing through long COVID-19. One will not be able to achieve optimal health, productivity and career progression if the amount of sleep that is being obtained.

EXERCISE

Exercise is preached about by everyone, however, it is rare that one will take the concept of exercise and directly relate it to an individual's routine. This becomes of great importance especially within the long COVID-19 context. Exercise is more than just the movement of your body to burn calories and build muscle. Exercise is a holistic approach towards a positive sense of health and wellbeing, focussing on adding more health benefits on a physical, mental and emotional scale.

Biologically, exercise plays an important role in the ability of our brains to deal with stress. There is an increase in the sensitivity to serotonin, which aids in the relief of symptoms that are associated with depression. Exercise further increases the presence of endorphins, promoting positivity and even reducing the sensations that are associated with pain.

Naturally, exercise aids in the support of a fast metabolism, making sure that the amount of calories that are being burned during the day is increased. Although we know that there is an increase in muscle mass that is associated with intense exercise, we need to relate this to the long COVID-19 context. As individuals who have long COVID-19 begin to exercise, they will need to strengthen their muscles and bones. This is why it is recommended that those that are progressing through long COVID-19, perform exercises that are non-weight bearing.

With individuals that suffer from chronic fatigue as well as the after-effects of long COVID-19, performing light to moderate amounts of exercise will increase the energy levels that you have, allowing you to fill your day up with important tasks that need to be completed. Ultimately, regular physical activity will help you sleep better. It doesn't matter whether the exercise is aerobic or resistance training, exercise is exercise.

What we see is that exercise has the potential to influence most of the domains of our lives, allowing us to have a more positive approach towards life. In the context of long COVID-19, exercise will aid in the production of hormones that make you sleep better, improving your skin's appearance and decreasing the chances of you developing a chronic disease. The fact remains, exercise in moderate doses will impact your life in a positive way.

The R.I.S.E protocol is a detailed approach that allows you to take ownership of your life after long COVID-19. It further allows you to reintegrate yourself back into society within a phased manner that does not place any unrealistic expectations on you. Having successfully overcome COVID-19 as well as long COVID-19 you are seen as a force to be reckoned with. Through following the R.I.S.E protocol through this time, you will be able to effectively motivate yourself to get back on track towards your optimal state of health.

CONCLUSION

Long COVID-19 has proven to be a severe complication of COVID-19. With many healthcare professionals remaining confused regarding what it entails, as far as we know the most that we can do is remain healthy, provide emotional support and exercise when we can. What we know for certain is that long COVID-19 is real and has the potential to really turn somebody's life upside down. We have read the stories from those that have gone through the recovery process, and what we know for sure is that long COVID-19 is serious.

What we wanted to do was make sure you are equipped for any form of symptom that may come your way due to long COVID-19, as well as allow you to relay information to others that may be going through the same recovery process. Catering for different people and their preferences is not easy however, being equipped with treatments, alternative therapies and self-help options, we believe that there is enough information to ensure that you are able to cope effectively with long COVID-19 and overcome this post-viral illness.

The impact and effect that adequate nutrition and supplementation has on your recovery process should not be overlooked. Many a time we prefer the quick fix meals, whether it be greasy or rather unhealthy for us. However, taking some extra time to write a shopping list with nutritious foods, will make the world of difference. Nutrition is important, and is to be prioritized in cases such as long COVID-19.

A very important aspect that we touched on was the effects of anxiety, stress and depression during this time of long COVID-19. We find that being isolated has such a great toll on our mental health, that it is difficult to combat both that as well as a post-viral illness. We emphasized the recommendation of a support group because realistically, long COVID-19 is not acknowledged as being important. However, the online community that is directly associated with long COVID-19 in terms of being survivors of the post-viral illness, have banded together in order to educate and empower those that are struggling through long COVID-19.

The depression that is associated with long COVID-19, as well as the negative spirals that can be initiated may be difficult to control however, we have full faith that using the resources that you have obtained in this book that you will be able to make that mental shift towards a more positive outlook both during and after long COVID-19.

There are so many different types of apps and audiobooks that are available in order to ensure that you are taking effective mindfulness breaks and that you are focusing on your mental wellbeing. It may be difficult at the beginning, but trust us when we say that it will get easier with time. What you need to focus on is yourself, your goals as well as ensuring that you recover fully from long COVID-19.

We are not saying that it is going to be an easy journey because it never really is. However, what we want to ensure is that you know that there is an end of the tunnel, and that it may feel like you are going through this recovery alone. However, there are loved ones that care for you and want to make sure that you are healthy again. We know and acknowledge that things may be tough at home however, you are tougher and stronger than any disease.

Deciding to return to the normal world may also pose some difficulties. One becomes so scared of not only what others think, but we also start to lose trust in our own capabilities. Sometimes we will falter, other times we will feel as though we are the most positive individuals on the planet. What we really want you to know is that long COVID-19 can be managed, you can and will be able to work again, and know your life is not over. Your life is only just beginning, and as soon as you overcome this hurdle of long COVID-19, you will be well on your way to success.

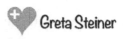 Greta Steiner

GET THE EXTRAS!

R.I.S.E. Protocol®
Diet Plans & Nutrition Guide

Facebook Group
to return to health

By Greta Steiner

REFERENCES

Altered sensations. (n.d.). MS Trust. Retrieved August 30, 2020, from https://www.mstrust.org.uk/a-z/altered-sensations#:~:text=Paraesthesia%3A%20an%20annoying%20unusual%20sensation

Chest burning: Causes, treatments, and home remedies. (2019, September 6). Www.Medicalnewstoday.Com. https://www.medicalnewstoday.com/articles/326273#when-to-see-a-doctor

COVID-19: How countries were affected and how governments responded. (2020, April 24). People's Assembly. https://www.pa.org.za/blog/covid-19-how-countries-were-affected-and-how-gover

DeSarkisson, C. (2018, November 25). *Causes of Tingling in Hands and Feet.* WebMD. https://www.webmd.com/brain/tingling-in-hands-and-feet#3-5

Fatigue Causes. (2020, July 20). Mayo Clinic. https://www.mayoclinic.org/symptoms/fatigue/basics/causes/sym-20050894#:~:text=Most%20of%20the%20time%20fatigue

Garner, P. (2020, May 5). *Paul Garner: For 7 weeks I have been through a roller coaster of ill health, extreme emotions, and utter exhaustion.* The BMJ. https://blogs.bmj.com/bmj/2020/05/05/paul-garner-people-who-have-a-more-protracted-illness-need-help-to-understand-and-cope-with-the-constantly-shifting-bizarre-symptoms/

How family and friends can help. (2018, January 29). Marie Curie. https://www.mariecurie.org.uk/help/support/being-there/helping-someone-cope/family-friends-help

Mahase, E. (2020). Covid-19: What do we know about "long covid"? *BMJ*, m2815. https://doi.org/10.1136/bmj.m2815

Managing long-term illness and chronic conditions. (2012). Vic.Gov.Au. https://www.betterhealth.vic.gov.au/health/ServicesAndSupport/managing-long-term-illness-and-chronic-conditions

Most multivitamins and supplements are a "waste of money." (2018, May 29). Nhs.Uk. https://www.nhs.uk/news/medical-practice/most-multivitamins-and-supplements-are-waste-money/

NHS Choices. (2019a). *Bodybuilding and sports supplements: the facts - Healthy body.* https://www.nhs.uk/live-well/healthy-body/body-building-sports-supplements-facts/

NHS Choices. (2019b). *Moodzone.* https://www.nhs.uk/conditions/stress-anxiety-depression/coping-with-financial-worries/

NHS Choices. (2019c). *Moodzone.* https://www.nhs.uk/conditions/stress-anxiety-depression/coping-with-financial-worries/

Oran, D. (2020, June 17). *Up to 45% of covid infections may be asymptomatic — Scripps analysis.* Medical Brief. https://www.medical-brief.co.za/archives/up-to-45-of-covid-infections-may-be-asymptomatic-scripps-analysis/

Rascon, G. (2019, July 16). *What is Brain Fog? Symptoms & Treatment Options.* SteadyMD. https://www.steadymd.com/2019/07/16/brain-fog/#:~:text=Brain%20fog%20is%20the%20inability

Recovering from COVID-19: Post viral-fatigue and conserving energy - RCOT. (n.d.). Www.Rcot.Co.Uk. Retrieved September 2, 2020, from https://www.rcot.co.uk/recovering-covid-19-post-viral-fatigue-and-conserving-energy

Stress and Addiction. (2012). Matt Gonzales. Drug Rehab. https://www.drugrehab.com/recovery/dealing-with-stress/

Made in the USA
Las Vegas, NV
02 May 2024

89403658R00080